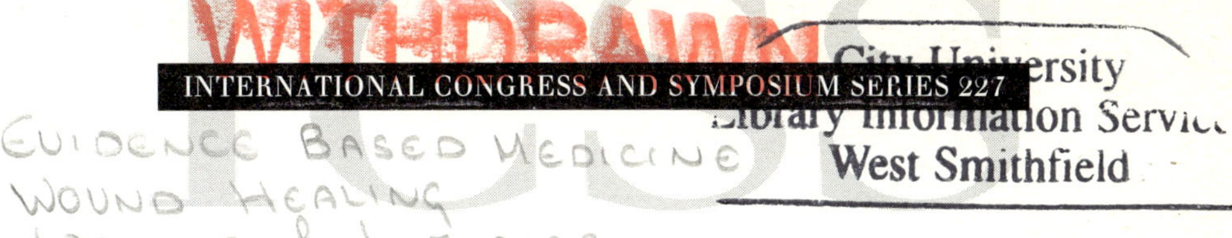

INTERNATIONAL CONGRESS AND SYMPOSIUM SERIES 227

Editor-in-Chief: Lord Walton of Detchant

Evidence-based woundcare

Edited by

A Suggett, G Cherry, R Mani, W Eaglstein

Proceedings of a conference sponsored by Smith & Nephew held in York, UK on 17th November 1997

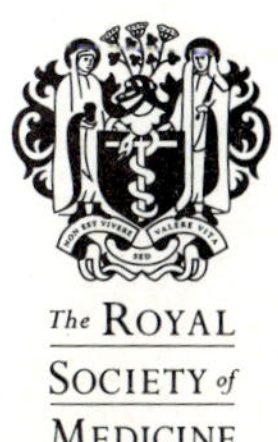

The ROYAL SOCIETY of MEDICINE PRESS Limited

INTERNATIONAL CONGRESS AND SYMPOSIUM SERIES 227

1 Wimpole Street, London, W1M 8AE, UK
16 East 69th Street, New York, NY 10021, USA

These proceedings are published by Royal Society of Medicine Press Ltd with financial support from the sponsor. The contributors are responsible for the scientific content and for the views expressed, which are not necessarily those of the sponsor, of the editor of the series or of the volume, of the Royal Society of Medicine or of the Royal Society of Medicine Press Ltd. Distribution has been in accordance with the wishes of the sponsors but a copy is available to any fellow of the Society at a privileged price.

British Library Cataloguing in Publication Data
A catalogue record for this book is available from the British Library
ISBN 1-85315-349-4
ISSN 0142-2367

Phototypeset by Dobbie Typesetting Limited, Tavistock, Devon
Printed in Great Britain by Ebenezer Baylis, The Trinity Press, Worcester

INTERNATIONAL CONGRESS AND SYMPOSIUM SERIES 227

Participants

EDITORS

Professor A Suggett
SMITH & NEPHEW GROUP RESEARCH CENTRE, YORK SCIENCE PARK, HESLINGTON, YORK YO1 5DF

Dr G Cherry
OXFORD WOUND HEALING INSTITUTE, DEPARTMENT OF DERMATOLOGY, CHURCHILL HOSPITAL, HEADINGTON, OXFORD WX3 7LJ

Dr R Mani
DEPARTMENT OF MEDICAL PHYSICS AND BIOENGINEERING, MAIL POINT 29, SOUTHAMPTON UNIVERSITY HOSPITAL NHS TRUST, TREMONA ROAD, SOUTHAMPTON SO16 6YD

Professor W Eaglstein
DEPARTMENT OF DERMATOLOGY AND CUTANEOUS SURGERY, UNIVERSITY OF MIAMI, SCHOOL OF MEDICINE, PO BOX 016259 (R-250), MIAMI, FLORIDA 33010, USA

SPEAKERS

Dr PC Bauling
SPECIALIST SURGEON, 205 MEDFORUM, 412 SCHOEMAN STR, PRETORIA 0002 SOUTH AFRICA

Mrs M Benbow
MID CHESHIRE HOSPITALS TRUST, LEIGHTON HOSPITAL, CREWE, CHESHIRE CW1 4QJ, UK

Mrs A Foster
KING'S COLLEGE HOSPITAL, DENMARK HILL, LONDON SE5 9RS, UK

Professor K Harding
WOUND HEALING RESEARCH UNIT, DEPARTMENT OF SURGERY, UNIVERSITY OF WALES COLLEGE OF MEDICINE, CARDIFF CF4 4XN, UK

Dr M Leek
MANCHESTER BIOTECH LTD, 3.239 STAPFORD BUILDING, OXFORD ROAD, MANCHESTER M13 9PT, UK

Dr L Martini
PLASTIC SURGERY DIVISION, OESPEDALE SANTA MARIA ANNUNZIATA, VIA DI ANTELLA, 58, 50011 ANTELLA (FI), ITALY

Dr J Posnett
YORK HEALTH ECONOMICS CONSORTIUM, UNIVERSITY OF YORK, HESLINGTON, YORK YO1 5DD, UK

SPEAKERS
(continued)

Dr P Price
WOUND HEALING RESEARCH UNIT, DEPARTMENT OF SURGERY, UNIVERSITY OF WALES COLLEGE OF MEDICINE, CARDIFF CF4 4XN, UK

Dr E Ricci
DEPARTMENT OF VULNOLOGY, NEW S. PAUL CLINIC, TURIN, ITALY

Dr M Richardson
SMITH & NEPHEW WOUND MANAGEMENT DIVISION, PO BOX 81, HESSLE ROAD, HULL HU3 2BN, UK

Dr J Rose
SMITH & NEPHEW GROUP RESEARCH CENTRE, YORK SCIENCE PARK, HESLINGTON, YORK YO1 5DF, UK

Dr M Romanelli
DEPARTMENT OF DERMATOLOGY, UNIVERSITY OF PISA, VIA ROMA 67, 56126 PISA, ITALY

Dr R Sibbald
UNIVERSITY OF TORONTO, SUITE BW4-658, 585 UNIVERSITY AVENUE, TORONTO, ONTARIO, CANADA M5G 2C4

Dr N Shioya
WOUNDCARE HEALING CENTRE, KITASATO UNIVERSITY SCHOOL OF MEDICINE, MINATO-KU, TOKYO, JAPAN

Dr M Stacey
DEPARTMENT OF SURGERY, THE UNIVERSITY OF WESTERN AUSTRALIA, FREMANTLE HOSPITAL, GPO BOX 480, FREMANTLE, WESTERN AUSTRALIA 6160, AUSTRALIA

Contents

Contents

(continued)

Contents

(continued)

Session 5:

CLINICAL EVIDENCE OF COST-EFFECTIVENESS

Session 6:

WOUNDCARE INTO THE MILLENNIUM

Foreword

The first symposium on Evidence-based woundcare was held in York on Sunday 16 and Monday 17 November 1997. With the development of new technologies, woundcare management has reached a very exciting stage, with many implications for the present and future management of wounds.

The meeting drew together an international team of experts — Professor William Eaglstein (University of Miami), Dr Raj Mani (Southampton University Hospitals Trust), Dr George Cherry (Oxford Wound Healing Institute) and Professor Alan Suggett (Group Research Director, Smith & Nephew) — from a variety of disciplines to address a diverse range of issues.

Session 1
WOUND HEALING

A review of moist wound healing

W EAGLSTEIN

DEPARTMENT OF DERMATOLOGY AND CUTANEOUS SURGERY,
UNIVERSITY OF MIAMI SCHOOL OF MEDICINE, MIAMI, FLORIDA, USA

Within the last decade moist wound healing (MWH) has become a mainstream of medical practice and there are now about 1000 different occlusive dressings, most aimed at producing MWH. The Smith Papyrus of 1615 BC noted that wounds closed faster in the moist environment created by gum-impregnated linen strips. Hippocrates, in contrast, advised leaving wounds open to relieve bad humours. Until the 19th century, drainage continued to be encouraged, as illustrated by the phrase, 'laudable pus'. Lister's work led to an obsessive fear of pus as an indication of infection. Since occlusive dressings are often associated with an accumulation of neutrophil-containing wound fluid, the strong linkage between pus and infection prevented and still inhibits the use of occlusion to obtain moist wound healing.

In 1948, Oscar Gilje's thesis documented the favourable 'moist chamber effect' of adhesive tape occlusion for leg ulcers[(1)]. In 1950 Schilling *et al* compared occlusive, semi-occlusive and open therapy of minor injuries[(2)]; unfortunately they emphasized the negative effects of complete occlusion and overlooked the beneficial effects of semi-occlusive therapy. Nevertheless in 1951 Beattie *et al*, wanting to inspect wounds without removing dressings, published papers on nearly 300 cases of abdominal and thoracic surgery treated with a plastic film 'window-pane' dressing[(3)]. No infections occurred. By 1958 Odland found that induced friction blisters left intact healed faster when covered than when uncovered[(4)]. The 1962 work of Winter, showing that resurfacing beneath occlusion in superficial pig wounds was approximately 30% faster than in open conditions, is usually cited as the key piece of experimental work in the MWH literature[(5)]. Hinman and Maibach then demonstrated the same effect in human wounds[(6)]. The difficulties to be encountered in establishing occlusive dressing therapy were foreshadowed in their closing paragraph, which noted that '... perhaps with the introduction of potent anti-microbial agents for the skin, it might now be practical

EVIDENCE-BASED WOUNDCARE, EDITED BY A SUGGETT, G CHERRY, R MANI, W EAGLSTEIN, 1998.
INTERNATIONAL CONGRESS AND SYMPOSIUM SERIES NO 227 PUBLISHED BY THE ROYAL SOCIETY OF MEDICINE PRESS LIMITED

to take advantage of an occlusive dressing'. Linsky *et al*[7], were among the first to document the dermal effects of occlusion.

Despite scientifically-based literature on the benefits of MWH, including wound healing model results published in 1978[8], the fear that occlusive dressings would induce infection precluded their use. It was largely due to nurses that they finally entered the market. Nurses began covering chronic wounds with materials such as Incise Drape, designed to be placed over incision sites to prevent bacteria from migrating into surgical incisions and their anecdotal reports of the beneficial effects of these films and stomal adhesives ultimately convinced companies to make occlusive dressings[9,10].

In the late 1970s the first occlusive dressing, Opsite (Smith & Nephew) was introduced. Several years later the first hydrocolloid, variously known as Granuflex or DuoDerm, was introduced, based on a product called Stomadhesive, used in ileostomy management. But occlusive dressings still encountered considerable resistance, especially from physicians[11]. They were often associated with a suppurative wound fluid and foul odours — due to wound proteases acting on the gelatin and pectin of the dressing — and ran counter to the notion of avoiding infections by letting wounds dry.

In 1985 Mertz *et al*[12] suggested that occlusive therapy may actually prevent wound infections, by excluding pathogens from the wound site. Hutchinson's 1989 compilation[13] was particularly compelling, demonstrating that the chance of infection under occlusion was 2.6% compared to 7.1% with conventional therapy. There is now a substantial body of studies showing that the chances of infection with occlusion are less than with conventional therapy[14–16]. By 1993, Brown and Zitelli had included the use of occlusive therapy in their guidelines for acute wound management[17] and, in 1994, a panel created by the US Agency for Healthcare Policy Research, led by Bergstrom, recommended MWH in their US Guidelines for the Treatment of Pressure Ulcers[18].

This history of MWH and occlusive dressings offers many general lessons, including that:

- intuition can be misleading — allowing wounds to dry is intuitive, but counter-productive
- often rules do not apply universally — increased moisture and bacteria have not led to increased infections
- the creation of new information does not always produce a change in medical behaviour
- MWH has demonstrated that healing can be improved beyond its physiological state.

References

1 Gilje O. On taping (adhesive tape treatment) of leg ulcers. *Acta Derm Vener* 1948; **28**: 454–67.

2 Schilling RS, Roberts M, Lond M, Goodman N. Clinical trial of occlusive plastic dressings. *Lancet* 1950; **250**: 293–6.

3 Beattie AD, Dodd H, Nixon WC. A post-operative dressing. *Lancet* 1951; **14**: 816–17.

4 Odland G. The fine structure of the interrelationship of cells in the human epidermis. *J Biophy Biochem Cytol* 1958; **4**: 529–35.

5 Winter GD. Formation of scab and the rate of epithelization of superficial wounds in the skin of the young domestic pig. *Nature* 1962; **193**: 293–4.

6 Hinman CD, Maibach H. Effect of air exposure and occlusion on experimental human skin wounds. *Nature* 1963; **200**: 377–8.

7 Linsky CB, Rovee DT, Dow T. Effect of wound dressing on wound inflammation and scar tissue. In: Dineen P, ed. *The Surgical Wound.* Philadelphia: Lea and Febiger, 1981: 191–206.

8 Eaglstein WH, Mertz PM. New method for assessing epidermal wound healing: the effects of triamcinolone acetonide and polyethylene film occlusion. *J Invest Dermatol* 1978; **71**: 382–4.

9 Baum ME. Flexible decubitus treatment. *Nursing Care* 1976; July: 24–25.

10 Leeson M. Better decubitus care. *Nursing* 1976: 13.

11 Bennett RG. The debatable benefit of occlusive dressings for wounds. *Derm Surg Oncol* 1982; **8**: 166–7.

12 Mertz PM, Marshall DA, Eaglstein WH. Occlusive wound dressings to prevent bacterial invasion and wound infection. *J Am Acad Dermatol* 1985; **12**: 662–8.

13 Hutchinson JJ. Prevalence of wound infection under occlusive dressings: a collective survey of reported research. *Wounds* 1989; **1**: 123–33.

14 Hulton L. Dressings for surgical wounds. *Am J Surg* 1994; **167**(suppl): 42S–45S.

15 Smith DJ. Microbiology and healing of occluded skin graft donor sites. *Plast Recon Surgery* 1993; **91**: 1094–7.

16 Rubio PA. Use of semiocclusive, transparent film dressings for surgical wound protection: experience in 3637 cases. *Int Surg* 1991; **76**: 253–4.

17 Brown CD, Zitelli JA. Acute wound management guidelines. *J Derm Surg Oncol* 1993; **19**: 732–7.

18 Bergstrom N, Bennett MA, Carlson CE, *et al.* Treatment of pressure ulcers. Clinical Practice Guideline, No 15. Rockville, MD: US Department of Health and Human Services. Public Health Service, Agency for Health Care Policy and Research. AHCPR Publication No 95-0652. December 1994.

The microenvironment around leg ulcers

R MANI, L HAMMAD AND G ROBERTS

DEPARTMENT OF MEDICAL PHYSICS AND BIOENGINEERING,
SOUTHAMPTON GENERAL HOSPITAL, UK

Since the seminal studies of George Winter that led to the development of occlusive dressings, it has become accepted that a moist environment favours healing. Such an environment is engendered by dressings that absorb wound exudates while keeping the wound bed moist. Leaving a wound open causes it to dry, generating conditions that are less favourable to healing. The purpose of this paper is to examine how moist wound dressings influence the microenvironment in which healing occurs.

A reasonable definition of microenvironment might be the milieu in which healing occurs: the physiological and biochemical parameters involved in the process are the key host players, while infection is the key foreign one. Wound healing is a vast subject and — for the purposes of this discussion — only chronic wounds will be considered, of which leg ulcers, diabetic foot ulcers and pressure sores are the best examples. This paper will also examine reliable methodology for determining some of the physical changes within wounds.

Chronic wounds

Venous ulcers are the most common type of leg ulcer, affecting 3% of the elderly and consuming up to £400m annually in the UK[1]. Diabetic foot ulcers cost even more and cost-considerations alone make chronic wound healing an important issue. The discomfort, pain and loss of work are arguably more important however, and must also be taken into account. Pressure sores and head and neck wounds resulting from radionecrosis are also difficult to manage; the need exists for an optimal healing environment.

EVIDENCE-BASED WOUNDCARE, EDITED BY A SUGGETT, G CHERRY, R MANI, W EAGLSTEIN, 1998.
INTERNATIONAL CONGRESS AND SYMPOSIUM SERIES NO 227 PUBLISHED BY THE ROYAL SOCIETY OF MEDICINE PRESS LIMITED

What signifies reliable healing? As granulation occurs and fresh epithelium grows over the open surface, the wound is considered to be responding to treatment. Decreasing contour dimensions and photographs may partially satisfy our need for evidence of the healing of surface wounds. With deep wounds, the extent of dermal invasion must be assessed; this may be complicated by the undermining at the edge of the wound evident when ulcers are debrided surgically. The speed of the wound-healing response varies during the healing process, with systemic illness, wound infection and uncontrolled oedema all modulating wound response to treatment. Poor compliance must also be considered; some centres include patients' attitudes to treatment in quality of life appraisals. Physiological parameters such as nutrition are also central to healing.

Physiological parameters of healing

Tissue nutrition

Tissue nutrition must be sufficient to promote angiogenesis and epithelialization and to defend the host against infection. Angiogenesis is promoted in hypoxic environments; capillaries grow along decreasing gradients of oxygen tension[(2)]. The tissues surrounding venous ulcers are hypoxic[(3)], despite satisfactory levels of perfusion[(4)]. Francek proposed that diminished capillary density was responsible for local hypoxia[(5)] and used a tissue oxygen probe with an inbuilt microscope that allowed capillaries in the test site to be counted. However his proposal contradicted observations that sites of atrophie blanche rarely ulcerate. The density of capillaries in peripheral tissues varies with prolonged venous hypertension; most claim it decreases[(6)], although others claim it increases[(7)]. Other morphological changes observed in capillaries by Mourad[(7)] include an increased endothelial luminal volume which favours increased permeability.

Changes triggered by increased retrograde venous pressures include increased vascular permeability and loss of pre-capillary sphincter control, which in turn promotes oedema formation. There is evidence that oedema impedes healing[(8)]. Barnes examined the effects of bed elevation on leg oedema and found that significant decreases in leg volumes were associated with statistically significant increases in tissue perfusion[(9)]. He used a laser Doppler and tissue oxygen electrodes to measure microvascular flow and skin oxygen tension in 13 patients with chronic venous ulcers and very swollen, unmanageable legs. Control measurements on ipsilateral forearms did not alter significantly during this period. It is likely that decreasing afterload caused a decrease in tissue pressure with concomitant increase in tissue nutrition parameters. This is similar to the observations of increased tissue oxygen levels associated with decreased oedema, following treatment with sequential intermittent compression[10,11]. These reports suggest that oedema may impede oxygen diffusion in peripheral tissues[3].

Tissue oxygen and blood flow measurements

Tissue oxygen may be measured invasively, or non-invasively[12] using the transcutaneous probe devised by Huch. Tissue oxygen measurements indicate clearly that tissues vulnerable to ulceration are hypoxic. The role of hypoxia is paradoxical; it promotes angiogenesis, possibly mediated by macrophages, but also favours the growth of fibroblasts within narrow 'windows' of tissue oxygen levels. Macrophage activity is thought to produce growth factors such as epidermal growth factor (EGF), platelet derived growth factor (PDGF) and transforming growth factors (TGF) some of which are presumed to be turned off once a repair is complete.

Through their effects on fibroblasts, it is suggested that hypoxic media promote the synthesis and transcription of at least one growth factor, namely TGF(β_1)[13]. Fibroblast activity is essential for the development of the collagen matrix, another basic substrate for tissue to grow on. It therefore seems likely that other physical properties of the medium may influence healing. Hunt proposed that pH could be critical in healing[14]; current evidence on pH in leg ulcers is discussed later in this paper.

At microvascular levels, blood flow may be reliably measured using a laser Doppler flowmeter — now available in different shapes and sizes, some extremely small — to measure flow in very small sample volumes[15]. Laser Doppler flowmetry may be used to demonstrate the postural control of the microcirculation — a local, sympathetic response that is mediated neurally and considered to offer protection from oedema formation[16]. Laser Doppler imaging, an advance on flowmetry, may be reliably used to measure the perfusion changes in full-thickness burn injuries.

In the diabetic patient, microvascular flow is normally higher at rest, but pathological changes within the vessels reduce their ability to vasodilate after a controlled ischeamic insult (reactive hyperaemia)[17]. This is easily demonstrated using a laser Doppler flowmeter and suggests why diabetic skin may be unable to meet the increased demands of the repair of ulceration and the frequency of ulceration of the diabetic foot.

Effects of oedema on periulcerous tissues

In the dependent position, the effects of high venous pressures are limited by the postural regulation mechanism. This phenomenon may be studied either by measuring swelling rates of the dependent extremity using strain gauge plethysmography or by measuring blood flow changes in the microcirculation using a laser Doppler flowmeter. In principle, an increase in hydrostatic pressure equivalent to 50 cm of water is counteracted by a decrease in blood flow. This reduction is achieved by reducing the radius of precapillary sphincters which provides protection against oedema formation[(18)] and is termed the arteriovenous response (AVR). The AVR may be detected at various sites on the leg and foot using a laser Doppler flowmeter; it is followed during passive lowering of the limb to 50 cm below heart level.

In our laboratory, a recent controlled study examined 15 patients with frank ulceration and 43 with venous insufficiency; there were 32 control subjects and all patients were aged between 21–81 [Unpublished data]. The study revealed that patients with frank ulceration have a clearly diminished AVR compared with patients who have venous pathology and control subjects. A lasting diminution of AVR in patients with frank ulcers is shown in Figure 1; also depicted is the decrease in laser Doppler response with leg lowering as a function of time in three groups. Hammad also carried out extensiometer measurements and found that in the presence of frank ulceration (and oedema), controlled stretching of the skin in the gaiter region has a lasting 'vasoconstrictor' effect as shown in Figure 2. In comparison, local

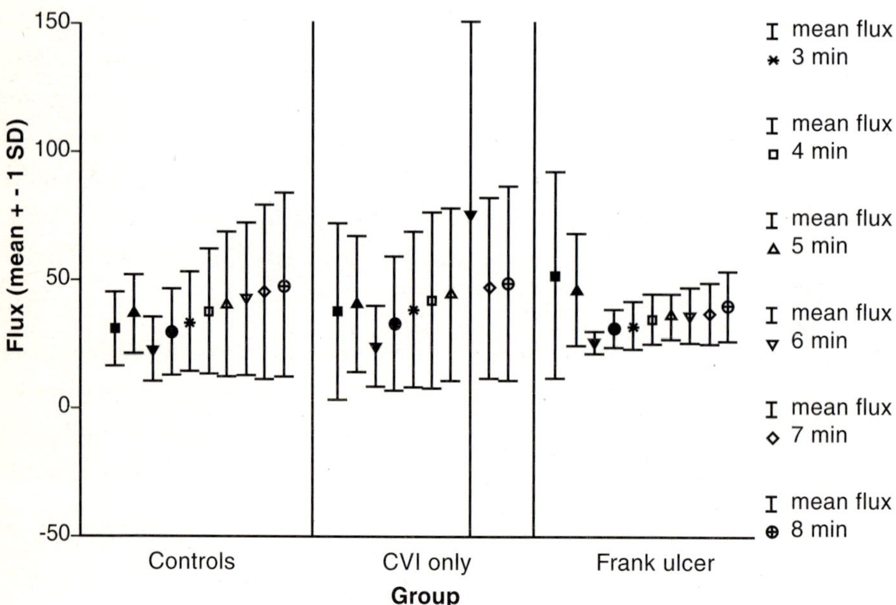

Figure 1

Change in laser Doppler flux with leg-lowering in controls, those with chronic venous insufficiency (CVI) only and those with frank ulcer

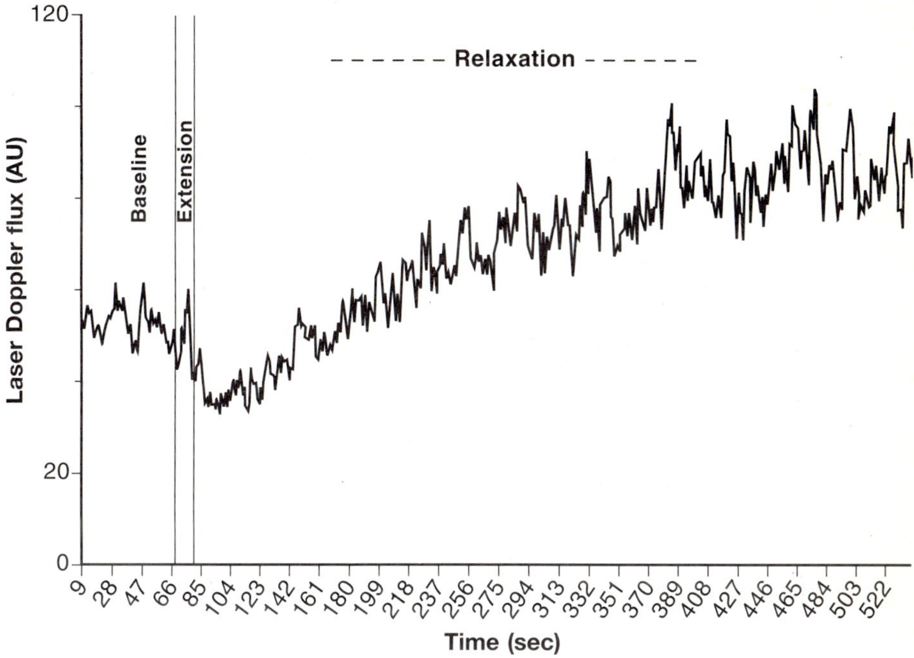

Figure 2

Laser Doppler blood flux during uniaxial extension

microvascular perfusion in healthy controls and patients with chronic venous insufficiency recovered rapidly, demonstrating a hyperaemic response.

These experiments suggest that the excess intestinal tissue pressures resulting from oedema may alter the normally visco-elastic properties of the gel matrix. To determine the effects of oedema it is necessary to locate it, and this can be achieved non-invasively using magnetic resonance imaging or ultrasound. The latter technique has the advantage of being simpler, less traumatic for the patient, and less expensive.

Ultrasound imaging

Gnaidecka and Serup demonstrated a simple method of quantifying the low echogenicity that is a feature of oedematous skin[(19)]. In Southampton, a high resolution ultrasound system has been developed that is capable of imaging as well as measuring stiffness (Figure 3). Typically the resolution of this system is around 100 microns.

To quantify some tissue properties, ultrasound echoes may be analysed. One method is to use the Fast Fourier Transform technique which determines the frequency content of an echo.

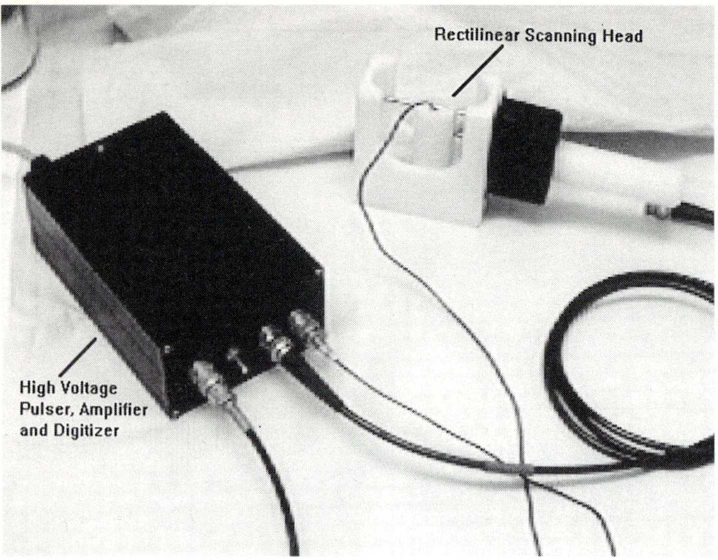

Figure 3

High voltage pulser, amplifier and digitizer, and rectilinear scanning head. The image may be displayed on a PC. The probe is held in a water bath

Ultrasound has been used to characterize thyroid and liver tissues in order to understand pathological processes. All images are visually characterized and experts are able to discriminate between pathological changes and normal tissues. With tissues vulnerable to ulceration, ultrasound characterization offers the only atraumatic method of determining physical properties such as stiffness and structure.

Does tissue structure break down?

It is accepted that, while most ulcers respond to treatment, a great number relapse. It may be that uncorrected venous hypertension will extort a high price from peripheral tissues. It is also possible that there is a problem with tissue structure in patients whose legs and ulcers deteriorate and a clue may lie in the exudate.

The fluid exudate from ulcers is unpleasant and often malodorous. When these fluids strike through the dressing covering the wound, they offer a passage for bacteria to invade the wound. No optimal method of sampling exudates exists, although analysis is relatively simple using pre-packaged radio-immunoassay kits. Cellulose sponges have the potential to soak wound exudates but Trentgrove and Stacey aspirated through a wound dressing[20]. In this study patients were fasted overnight, given a litre of water at 7 am and then asked to sit with legs dependent for an hour before fluid was drawn off using a hypodermic needle. The analysis revealed that chronic venous ulcers harbour a number of proteins and that inflammation markers are detectable in the fluid. Similar evidence of higher weight proteins in fluids have emerged from other centres. There is also some evidence that matrix metalloproteinase activity levels (MMP 2 and 9) are raised in chronic wound fluids[21].

In acute wounds there is clearly a need for clot formation to precede the repair process. In chronic wounds there may be an imbalance between the synthesis of collagen matrices and the degradation process affecting the structure and strength of tissues. These may be studied with ultrasound and other appropriate physical methods to determine an index of strength.

Determination of pH

Work carried out in our centre shows that surface pH may be measured reliably and non-invasively; the technique has been used in a study of patients with chronic venous ulcers being treated with the polyurethane foam dressing, Allevyn, and four-layer bandaging, Profore (both from Smith and Nephew)[22]. This study found that ulcer pH is significantly higher than control measurements on unbroken sites on the same limbs and that there is an association between acidity and healing. It is early days to look for predictive powers of pH measurements but the methodology is satisfactory and is recommended to develop better understanding of the healing environment (Figure 4).

Discussion

There is evidence that the microenvironment in moist wounds is well-perfused, but hypoxic. The regulation of microvascular flow is impaired and this will favour oedema formation. Work in our laboratory, in accord with the work of Romanelli *et al*[23], also indicates that acidity and healing are associated; acidification promotes healing.

Unrelieved oedema influences the microenvironment by affecting the microcirculation and impairing the viscoelastic properties of the gel matrix. Evidence from wound exudate studies suggest that both inflammatory mediators and matrix metalloproteinase activity are altered in

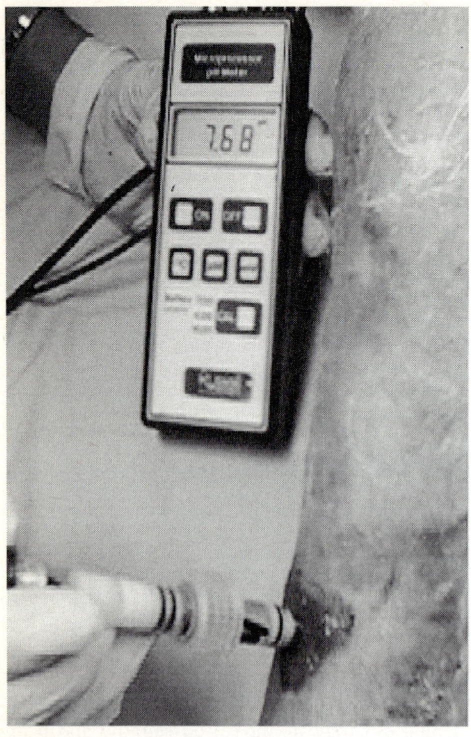

Figure 4

Measuring surface pH using a Russell glass electrode. A drop of de-ionized water is used to preserve contact with ulcer

the milieu of chronic ulcers, and it may be that there is some interdependence between these biochemical markers of tissue activity. There is a need to examine these biochemical markers together with physical indices of structure in developing a clear picture of the micro-environment in which healing occurs.

References

1 Fletcher A, Cullum N, Sheldon TA. A systematic review of compression treatment for venous ulcers. *BMJ* 1997; **315**: 576–80.

2 Remensnyder JP, Majno G. Oxygen gradients in healing wounds. *Am J Pathol* 1968; **52**: 301–8.

3 Mani R. Transcutaneous oxygen tension measurements in venous ulcer disease. *Vascular Med Rev* 1995; **6**: 121–31.

4 Sindrup JH, Arunsorp C, Steentos JH, Kristensen JK. Transcutaneous oxygen tension and laser Doppler flowmeter blood flow measurements in patients with venous ulcers. *Acta Dermatol Venerol* 1987; **67**(suppl): 160–82.

5 Francek U, Bollinger A, Huch R, Huch A. Transcutaneous oxygen tension measurements and capillary morphologic characteristics and density in patients with chronic venous insufficiency. *Circulation* 1984; **70**: 806–11.

6 Fagrell B. Local microcirculation in chronic venous insufficiency and leg ulcers. *Vascular Surg* 1979; **13**: 217–25.

7 Mourad MM, Barton SP, Marks R. Changes in endothelial mass, luminal volume and capillary numbers in the gravitational syndrome. *Br J Dermatol* 1992; **121**: 21–8.

8 Prasad AA, Ali Khan A, Mortimer PS. Leg ulcers and oedema; a study exploring the prevalence, aetiology and possible significance of oedema. *Phlebology* 1990; **5**: 181–7.

9 Barnes M, Mani R, White JE, Barrett DF. Changes in skin microcirculation during leg elevation in patients with chronic venous ulcers. *Phlebology* 1992; **7**: 36–9.

10 Olari PJ, Pekenmaki IK. Effects of intermittent compression treatment on skin perfusion and oxygenation of lower legs in venous ulcers. *VASA* 1987; **18**: 312–17.

11 Smith PC, Sarin S, Hasty J, Scurr JH. Sequential gradient pneumatic compression enhances venous ulcer healing: a randomised trial. *Surgery* 1990; **108**: 871–5.

12 Wyss CR, Matsen FA, Simmons CW, Burgess CM. Transcutaneous measurements of oxygen tension in limbs of diabetic and non-diabetic patients with peripheral vascular disease. *Surgery* 1984; **15**: 339–46.

13 Falanga V, Takagi H, Ceballos PI, Pardes JB. Low oxygen tension decreases receptor binding of peptide growth factors in dermal fibroblast cultures. *Exp Cell Res* 1994; **213**: 80–4.

14 Hunt TK. Wounds and wound healing. *Dis Colon Rectum* 1982; **25**: 1–15.

15 Sheppard A, Oberg P. *Laser Doppler flowmetry*. London: Kluwer Academic Publishers, 1990.

16 Hassan AA, Tooke JE. Effects of change in local skin temperature on postural vasoconstriction in man. *Clin Sci* 1988; **74**: 201–6.

17 Rayman G, Tooke JE. Impaired microvascular hyperemic response to minor skin trauma in type 1 diabetes. *BMJ* 1986; **292**: 1295–8.

18 Mani R. Venous haemodynamics: a consideration of macro and microvascular haemodynamics. *Proc Inst Mech Eng* 1992; **206**: 109–15.

19 Gnaidecka M, Quistorff B. Assessment of dermal water by high frequency ultrasound: comparative studies with nuclear magnetic resonance. *Br J Dermatol* 1996; **135**: 218–24.

20 Trentgrove N, Stacey M, McGechie S, *et al.* Qualitative bacteriology and leg ulcer healing. *J Wound Care* 1996; **5**: 277–80.

21 Wysocki A, Staino-Coico L, Grinelli F. Wound fluid from chronic leg ulcers contains elevated levels of metalloproteinases MMP2 and MMP9. *J Invest Dermatol* 1993; **10**: 64–8.

22 Glibbery A, Mani R. pH measurements in leg ulcers. *Int J Microcirc Clin Exptl* 1992; **109**(suppl).

23 Romanelli M, Schipani E, Piaggesi A, Barachini B. Evaluation of surface pH on venous leg ulcers under Allevyn dressings. In: Suggett A, Cherry G, Mani R, Eaglstein W, eds. *International Congress and Symposium Series No 227*. London: Royal Society of Medicine Press, 1998: 57–61.

Histology of wounds under dressings

M LEEK

MANCHESTER BIOTECH LTD, MANCHESTER, UK

The wound healing process represents a complex interaction between several cell types, each playing a specific role in a sequential cascade of events. The key stages to wound repair are: formation of a provisional matrix (clotting), followed by inflammation and proliferation of three different cell types:

- endothelial cells in the process of angiogenesis
- collagen fibril formation following fibroblast migration into the wound
- epithelialization — the resurfacing of the wound.

There then follow two more stages that have been relatively under-studied and are currently poorly understood — resolution and remodelling.

Histology of wound repair

Inflammation involves several different cell types. One of the first cell types to be seen are the neutrophils. Their main function is the killing of bacteria, but they also have a limited ability to phagocytose debris and bacteria that are present in the wound. They also produce a range of proteases which may be linked to the matrix breakdown, often observed in chronic wound formation[1]. Many studies into the role of neutrophils in wound healing have found that their depletion has little effect on the process.

The next inflammatory cell type is the macrophage. Until recently it was thought that macrophages had a single function, which was to phagocytose debris in the wound. Over the past five to six years it has been discovered that they actually orchestrate much of the healing

EVIDENCE-BASED WOUNDCARE, EDITED BY A SUGGETT, G CHERRY, R MANI, W EAGLSTEIN, 1998.
INTERNATIONAL CONGRESS AND SYMPOSIUM SERIES NO 227 PUBLISHED BY THE ROYAL SOCIETY OF MEDICINE PRESS LIMITED

process[2]. Macrophages are responsible for producing a range of different cytokines which up- and down-regulate different biological processes such as collagen formation. Dysfunctional macrophage populations within the wound may result in incomplete repair or the formation of chronic wounds.

An increasing number of lymphocytes begin to appear at the wound site at the same time as the macrophages. Little is understood about their role in wound healing, although recent publications have indicated that T lymphocytes may have some regulatory function, down-regulating some aspects of the repair process. Much remains to be learnt about the lymphocyte's role in wound healing. The purpose of angiogenesis is to establish a supply of oxygen and nutrients, and it involves endothelial cell migration into the wound. This is generally complemented by continued neo-matrix formation — fibroproliferation involves an influx of fibroblasts from the wound margins, followed by a secretion of collagen.

The late stages of the repair process involve resolution of fibroblasts and endothelial cells. The process is poorly understood and more research is required to establish the exact biological mechanisms involved. Dysfunctional resolution may lead to scarring complications such as keloids. The final stage is remodelling, in which the fibroblasts still left in the wound remodel the existing collagen to give it a higher tensile strength and integrity.

In some cases the interaction between cell types breaks down, leading to a dysfunctional repair process, culminating in chronic wound formation. Although the exact cause of wound chronicity is unclear in most cases, certain pathological features are consistent. These include excessive numbers of inflammatory cells, elevated protease levels and matrix deposition around vascular structures.

The influence of dressing type on the healing process

In an attempt to overcome some of the complications associated with the repair process, a diverse range of wound products has been developed. Wound dressings can be split into three broad categories:

- basic
- advanced, such as films, foams, hydrogels and hydrocolloids
- a group that can be termed 'bioactive', employing growth factors and tissue engineering.

Basic gauze is a very poor bacterial barrier and, because it is not occlusive, it allows the incorporation of foreign debris such as fibres into the wound. This also occurs with other types of dressing, although not with foams, such as Allevyn, or films, such as Opsite (both from Smith & Nephew). Foreign bodies evoke a strong reaction, involving granuloma formation, giant and other inflammatory cells.

Of the advanced products, films such as Opsite offer a good bacterial barrier, avoid incorporation of material into the wound, improve exudate control and create a moist environment which leads to faster epithelialization. There is also less damage on dressing removal. Advanced products, such as Allevyn foam, are able to control exudate much more effectively. Allevyn is very easy to remove from the surface of the wound, and some studies have shown that the cellular structure of the foam effectively draws bacteria and debris away from the surface of the lesion [Data on file. Smith & Nephew].

Gels such as Intrasite (Smith & Nephew) are very good at debriding necrotic material from the surface of chronic wounds and also provide very good exudate control. They may directly stimulate the repair process and some histological studies have shown that fragments of Intrasite gel interact with cells at the surface of the wound to stimulate macrophage function. Giant cells break down the dressing in a passive manner, there is no cell death and these cells may produce a range of cytokines which could actually stimulate the repair process.

Bioactive products will be on the market within the next five years. Growth factors will be used in the future to control the inflammatory cell profile of chronic wounds and this will hopefully overcome some of the dysfunction that is currently seen. There is also interest in manipulating growth factors to reduce fibrosis and thereby scarring[(3)].

Ongoing studies at Smith and Nephew have shown that some dysfunctional macrophages may contribute to the pathology seen in chronic wounds. In many wounds these cells are thought to have assumed an inappropriate phenotype, or in some cases may have become inactivated — having lost the ability to secrete the correct cytokine profile to initiate repair processes. By incubating such inactivated or dysfunctional cells with exogeneously applied macrophage stimulatory compounds it may be possible to start the repair process by pushing the cell into a more suitable phenotype. Cells stimulated in this way have been observed to produce a range of cytokines (such as transforming growth factor (TGF)-B, IL1, IL2, IL6 and platelet derived growth factor (PDGF)), many of which are intimately associated with modulation or regulation of the repair process; stimulation of such factors may help to overcome chronic wound pathology.

Tissue engineering will allow us to directly influence certain aspects of the repair process[(4)]. Adding fibroblastic, epidermal or endothelial components back into wounds may greatly speed up the healing of chronic lesions. With a cavernous wound, addition of a dermal replacement (or a dermal/epidermal replacement) should help to restore the tissue architecture. Furthermore, studies using materials such as Dermagraft [Data on file. Smith

& Nephew] and other tissue-engineered products have shown that the early application of fibroblastic cells to a lesion can reduce scarring.

Conclusion

Most, if not all, of the currently available woundcare products contribute to the repair process in some way, either by directly or indirectly altering cellular profiles[5]. As our understanding of the repair process and of dysfunctional elements increases, so will the number of products which are designed to directly modulate dysfunctional, cellular and biochemical processes within the lesion.

References

1 Herrick S, Ashcroft G, Ireland G, *et al.* Up-regulation of elastase in acute wounds of healthy aged humans and chronic venous leg ulcers are associated with matrix degradation. *Lab Invest* 1997; **77**(3): 281–8.

2 Leibovich SJ, Ross R. A macrophage-dependent factor that stimulates the proliferation of fibroblasts in vitro. *Am J Pathol* 1976; **84**: 501–14.

3 Shah M, Foreman DM, Ferguson MW. Neutralizing antibody to TGF-beta 1,2 reduces cutaneous scarring in adult rodents. *J Cell Sci* 1994; **107**: 1137–57.

4 Hansbrough JF, Morgan J, Greenleaf G, *et al.* Evaluation of Graftskin composite grafts on full-thickness wounds on athymic mice. *J Burn Care Rehabil* 1994; **15**: 346–53.

5 Harris B, Cai JP, Falanga V, *et al.* The effects of occlusive dressings on the recruitment of mononuclear cells by endothelial binding into acute wounds. *J Dermatol Surg Oncol* 1992; **18**: 279–83.

An adhesive hydrocellular dressing in the treatment of partial thickness skin graft donor sites

L MARTINI, UM REALI, L BORGOGNONI, P BRANDANI, A ANDRIESSEN

PLASTIC SURGERY DIVISION, SANTA MARIA ANNUNZIATA HOSPITAL, UNIVERSITY OF FLORENCE, ITALY

Partial thickness grafts are usually 300–375 μm thick. Donor sites traditionally dressed with paraffin gauze have a healing time of between seven and 12 days[1]. There are, however, some typical disadvantages observed with this dressing regime: adherence of the dressing to the wound bed — due to coagulation, damage and frictional trauma — and pain upon dressing removal[2]. Allevyn Adhesive hydrocellular dressing (Smith & Nephew) has been shown to be effective in the treatment of various wound types; this suggests that improvements could also be made in the treatment of donor sites[3,4].

The purpose of this study was to evaluate and compare the performance of the hydrocellular dressing, Allevyn, with a paraffin gauze dressing. The following factors were considered:

- time to complete epithelialization
- ease of dressing use
- pain on dressing removal
- cost-effectiveness of the dressing regime.

Methods

Fifty patients (28 women, 22 men) were enrolled in the study, of whom 44 were evaluated for end results. Patients' ages ranged from 18 to 88 years; mean 59.6. All grafts were taken from

EVIDENCE-BASED WOUNDCARE, EDITED BY A SUGGETT, G CHERRY, R MANI, W EAGLSTEIN, 1998.
INTERNATIONAL CONGRESS AND SYMPOSIUM SERIES NO 227 PUBLISHED BY THE ROYAL SOCIETY OF MEDICINE PRESS LIMITED

the thigh and harvested as partial thickness skin grafts using a manual dermatome. The size of the donor site ranged from 20 cm^2 to 71 cm^2; mean 43.4 cm^2. In each patient 50% of the donor site was covered with the hydrocellular dressing and 50% was covered with the paraffin gauze.

Upon each initial random dressing removal the patient was asked to rate the pain by giving a single mark on a 10 cm linear scale ranging from 'no pain' (0 cm) to 'pain I cannot bear' (10 cm). In order not to skew the pain assessment the dressing that did not adhere was removed first.

Results

Upon removal of the paraffin dressing all 44 patients scored 10 (pain I cannot bear). Upon removal of the hydrocellular dressing three patients scored 2 (slight pain) and 41 patients scored 0 (no pain).

After four days of treatment, the hydrocellular dressing was found to be easy to apply and remove. At the study endpoint (seven days), 41/44 patients had experienced complete epithelialization of this trial site—23 patients at four days, 18 at seven days and three at 10 days, with a mean time to complete epithelialization of 5.64 days, (SD $\pm$ 1.88).

In contrast, the paraffin gauze dressing had adhered completely to the wound bed in all 44 patients at four days, and was left in place. At day seven the paraffin gauze was still adhering to the wound bed in 28 patients, and dressing removal was not possible without causing damage to the wound bed. At the study endpoint (seven days), only 16/44 patients had experienced complete epithelialization of the trial site—26 at day 10 and two at day 12; mean nine days (SD $\pm$ 1.58).

Conclusion

The hydrocellular dressing demonstrated a significantly faster healing time than the paraffin gauze ($p < 0.01$). At day seven the trial site had completely epithelialized in 41 patients treated with paraffin gauze. The variance analysis for the overall healing time shows a significant difference in favour of the trial sites treated with hydrocellular dressing ($p < 0.000001$).

In six patients the section of the donor site dressed with paraffin gauze was infected and took up to 14 days to heal; in contrast, the section healed within four days. No infection occurred in the Allevyn site, suggesting that the risk of infection is reduced when using Allevyn Adhesive.

References

1 Hatz RA, Niedner R, Vanscheidt W, Westerhof W. *Wound healing and wound management*. Heidelberg: Springer-Verlag, 1994: 14–17.

2 Thomas S. Pain and wound management. *Nursing Times* 1989; **85**(suppl): 11–15.

3 Williams C, Young T. Allevyn Adhesive. *Br J Nurs* 1996; **3**: 691–3.

4 Kurring PA, Roberts CD, Quinlan D. Evaluation of a hydrocellular dressing in the management of exuding wounds in the community. *Br J Nurs* 1994; **3**: 1049–50.

Session 2
DESIGNING FOR CLINICAL NEEDS

Developing an advanced wound dressing

M RICHARDSON

SMITH AND NEPHEW WOUND MANAGEMENT DIVISION, HULL, UK

Any organization developing medical products needs to make patient/customer needs its main consideration. Technology can then be used to deliver the best solution to these needs within the appropriate regulatory framework. The application of technology without significant reference to customer needs is termed 'technology push', in contrast to 'technology pull', in which technology is harnessed in pursuit of customer benefits. Both approaches have advantages and disadvantages (Table 1). While 'technology push' challenges current thinking and can lead to major breakthroughs, if disengaged completely from customer needs, it can lead to products which struggle to find an application.

Satisfying wound management needs

With the growing acceptance of the moist wound healing (MWH) concept during the late 1970s it became clear that the technology and products available at the time were insufficient to achieve MWH in all wound types and stages of healing. It is interesting to reflect that, while at the time the MWH revolution was pioneered by film dressings such as Opsite (Smith & Nephew), we now view these as just a small part of the armoury.

Product designers were inspired to use materials and processing expertise to generate families of products that could assist in the achievement of MWH conditions(1). Many of the manufacturers made claims that individual products were the 'ideal wound dressing' for a wide variety of wounds and stages of healing. It soon became clear, however, that no single product or technology could deliver a universal MWH solution. Consequently a rational

EVIDENCE-BASED WOUNDCARE, EDITED BY A SUGGETT, G CHERRY, R MANI, W EAGLSTEIN, 1998.
INTERNATIONAL CONGRESS AND SYMPOSIUM SERIES NO 227 PUBLISHED BY THE ROYAL SOCIETY OF MEDICINE PRESS LIMITED

Table 1 Advantages and disadvantages of different technology approaches

	Technology Push	Technology Pull
Advantages	Challenges Current paradigms - breakthrough	- Driven by customer needs - Focuses and motivates development work
Disadvantages	- Lose sight of customer needs - Risk of 'product looking for application'	Miss major technology shifts

Push = lack of clearly defined need; Pull = clearly defined need

approach to product selection, based on proven performance and properties, was adopted[2]. Both clinical and scientific interest in wound management grew concurrently. Despite this, a variety of technologies and products continued to be developed and launched, often with limited supporting data. Some found a place within the armoury of the wound management clinicians and nurses, but others struggled.

The pharmaceutical industry, in partnership with customers, began to take a more educational approach and recognized that different products and technologies (eg alginates, films and foams) offered different benefits. Leading companies must recognize that, to have lasting success, a product development team must focus mainly on customer needs. Attractive technology on its own is valueless.

Identifying customer needs

When creating a new wound management product it is important to first, identify prospective customers and second, develop a clear understanding of their needs (Table 2). Identifying these needs is a complex task since the end patient or customer rarely has the opportunity to choose the product themselves. Although the impact a product has on their patients' wounds and quality of life will strongly influence the choice of the nurse or doctor, the products available to the clinician may also be limited by the product buyer.

Any development team needs to be sure that customer requirements are well-understood, defined and expressed in terms that are not 'solution-specific'. This means defining the unmet need rather than its perceived solution — for example a customer may say they require an adhesive-coated product when their real need is for a product that stays in place.

Table 2 *Key customers for a wound management product and their needs*

Customer	Needs
Patient	Quality of life
	Effectiveness
Nurse/clinician	Easy to use
	Cost-effective
	Evidence-based
	Reimbursement
	Proof
Buyer/payer	Low cost?
	Cost-effective
	Appropriate clinical endorsement
Others: The Government, carers, patients, family	

Satisfying customer needs

The constraints

All of us live and work in an environment with certain restrictions and constraints. Constraints also exist in the field of medical product development. It is important that all constraints are addressed and considered (Table 3) but, while developmental constraints exist for good reasons, they do not guarantee that products will meet customer needs. Products that add little or nothing to what is already available still often make it on to the market. Since failures are expensive, customer needs should remain paramount.

The process

A typical pre-launch product development pathway is shown in Figure 4. The whole process is focused on translating customer needs into product solutions using available technology.

Table 3 *The constraints that exist when developing wound management products*

What are the constraints?
• Environmental regulations — restricts materials/processes
• Design Control Regulations — FDA, EU
• GMP's — FDA, EU (manufacturing)
• Regulatory approval to sell — FDA, MDA, EU

Table 4 The product development process prior to launch

What is the process?	
1	Understand customer needs
2	Generate concepts
3	Create prototypes
4	Consult customers
5	Select preferred approach
6	Source technology (if not in-house)
7	Product stability, safety
8	Product efficacy (clinicals)
9	Process validation

Allevyn and Allevyn Adhesive (Smith & Nephew) were developed along this pathway; the need for a clean, MWH environment and the delivery of cost-effective care was achieved using advanced hydrocellular fluid handling technology, in combination with existing adhesive and film technology.

Conclusion

Understanding who our customers are and what their needs are is a complex field and it is vital that this is explored at the beginning of the design phase of a product. Designers need to guard against being so excited by new technology that they push it to market in the absence of a clear customer need (technology push). Product designers have to work in an environment constrained by regulations that exist to protect the customer. Although these regulations add cost and time to development, they reinforce the importance of prioritizing customer needs.

References

1 Thomas S. *Wound management and dressings.* London: The Pharmaceutical Press, 1990.

2 Turner TD. Which dressing and why? *Nursing Times* 1982; **29**(suppl): 1–3.

Effect of structure on the performance of a hydrocellular wound dressing

J ROSE

SMITH & NEPHEW GROUP RESEARCH CENTRE, YORK SCIENCE PARK, UK

Foam dressings are becoming important in the management of wounds. This paper looks at two such dressings — Allevyn (Smith & Nephew) and a competitor product — and relates their performance to the microstructure of the foams. Three properties of the dressings were tested:

- rate of absorbency
- fluid-retention properties
- pressure-relieving properties.

Experimental methods

The rate of absorbency was tested using a demand absorbency apparatus with no pressure gradient across the fluid-dressing interface, as described by Chatterjee[1]. The fluid-retention of the dressings was tested by immersing them until equilibrium was reached. They were then held over a measuring cylinder and the amount of fluid released from the dressing measured. The amount of fluid released was then calculated as a percentage of the total capacity of the saturated dressing.

The apparatus for measuring the pressure-relieving ability of a wound dressing is shown in Figure 1. The test method was designed to model pressure at the heel when a patient is resting in bed. The pressure gauge used was a Tally Scimedics Pressure Evaluator MKII with

EVIDENCE-BASED WOUNDCARE, EDITED BY A SUGGETT, G CHERRY, R MANI, W EAGLSTEIN, 1998.
INTERNATIONAL CONGRESS AND SYMPOSIUM SERIES NO 227 PUBLISHED BY THE ROYAL SOCIETY OF MEDICINE PRESS LIMITED

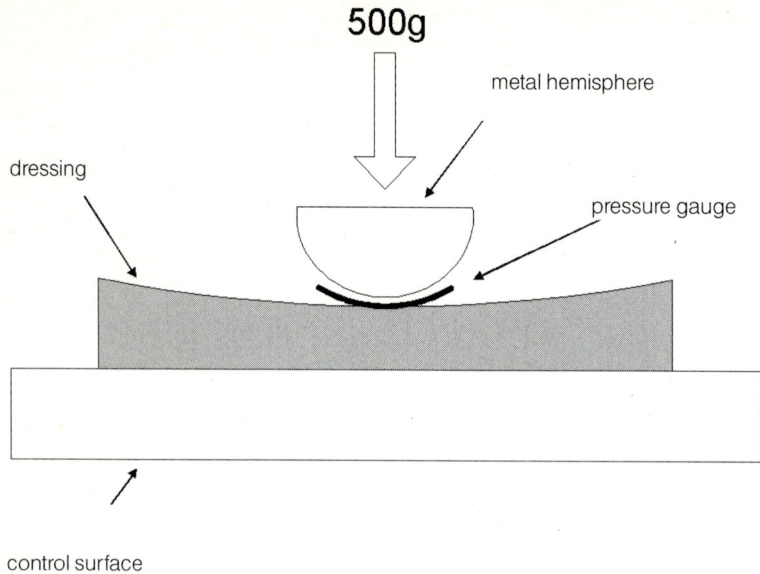

Figure 1

Schematic diagram of the method used to test the pressure-relieving ability of a wound dressing

a sensor diameter of 28 mm. The metal hemisphere diameter was 40 mm. Measurements were carried out on each dressing with a load of 500 g (Farrar has shown previously that 500 g corresponds to the load exerted at the heel in vivo[2] placed on the metal hemisphere). The measurement was repeated five times for each dressing and the average result applied to the following calculations. The pressure-relieving ability of the dressing was calculated as the difference in pressure with and without the sample, expressed as a percentage of the pressure measured without the sample.

Results

Two foams made from the same polymer (but with different cell sizes) were produced and tested for their rate of absorbency using the demand absorbency apparatus. The results are shown in Figure 2 and reveal that the polymer with the larger cell size reached saturation in approximately half the time. The fluid-retention test showed that Allevyn retained 93% of its saturated fluid while the competitor retained 28%. The pressure relief measurements showed that Allevyn provided a 17.4% relief in pressure, compared with 8.8% for the competitor product.

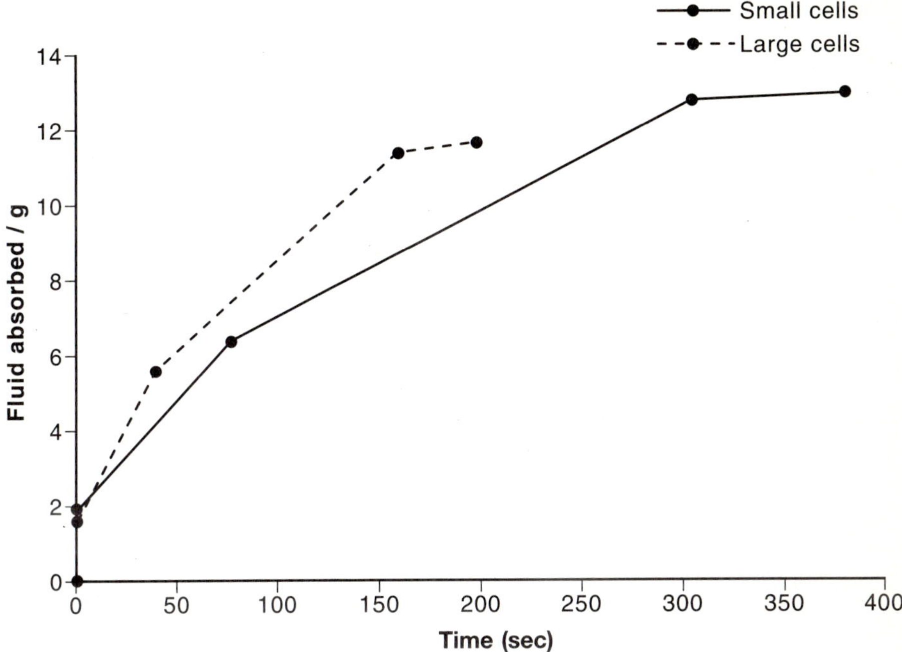

Figure 2

Graph showing the weight of fluid absorbed by foams with large and small cells as a function of time

Discussion and calculations

The results from the absorbency-rate testing show that there is an approximate factor of two difference in the saturation times of the two materials tested.

A cellular dressing may be modelled as a bundle of capillaries. The rate of fluid flow through a capillary is given by:

$$q = \frac{\pi P r^4}{8\eta l}$$

where q is the volume flux, r the capillary radius, η the fluid viscosity, l the length of the wetted capillary and P the pressure difference across the airliquid interface in the capillary[3,4]. The pressure difference can be written in terms of the capillary radius, r, thus:

$$P = \frac{2\gamma \cos\theta}{r}$$

In a capillary the fluid will eventually stop rising when a height, h, is reached. This height is related to the pressure by the following relationship:

$$P = \rho g h$$

If the ultimate height, h, is much greater than the thickness of the dressing, then the fluid flow rate will be approximately constant until the dressing is saturated. Finally, in a unit area there will be a number of capillaries, given by the following equation:

$$\text{number of capillaries} = \frac{1}{\pi r^2}$$

Overall the fluid flow rate for a dressing made of many capillaries is given by:

$$q = \frac{\pi r^4}{8\eta l} \cdot \frac{1}{\pi r^2} \cdot \frac{2\gamma \cos\theta}{r}$$

Assuming that 8, η, π, l, γ, $\cos\theta$ will be constant for a given polymer–liquid system, then the relationship simplifies to:

$$q \propto r$$

The cell sizes were measured as 100–150 microns and 200–250 microns for the two materials respectively. This is an approximate factor of two difference, therefore predicting a factor of two difference in the rate of absorption. This is reflected in the results, as the times to saturation are approximately 150 and 300 seconds, respectively.

The results of the fluid-retention test show that Allevyn retains more fluid than the competitor dressing, because of differences in structure. Again, using the capillary model, the height, h, to which a fluid will rise and the pressure difference across the air/fluid interface is important. Both properties are related to the capillary radius and simplifying the equation gives the following two relationships:

$$P \propto \frac{1}{r}$$

$$h \propto \frac{1}{r}$$

In other words, the smaller the capillary radius the higher, h, the fluid will rise and the greater the pressure, P, required to force the fluid out of the capillary. Relating this back to dressings, the smaller the cell size, the greater the pressure required to remove the fluid and the higher the fluid will track vertically. Thus dressings with smaller cell sizes will have better fluid-retention properties. Figure 3 shows SEM micrographs for the two dressings.

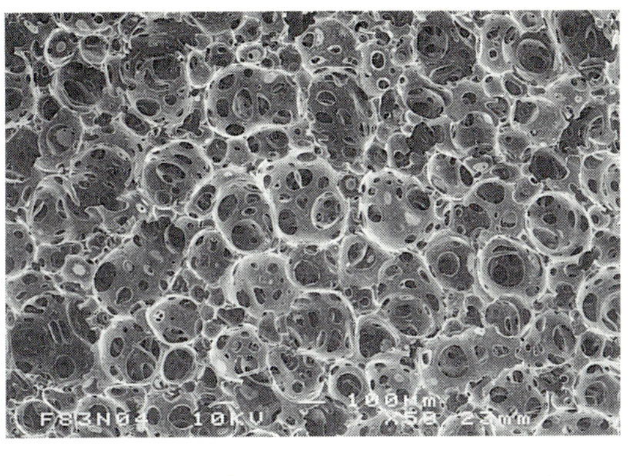

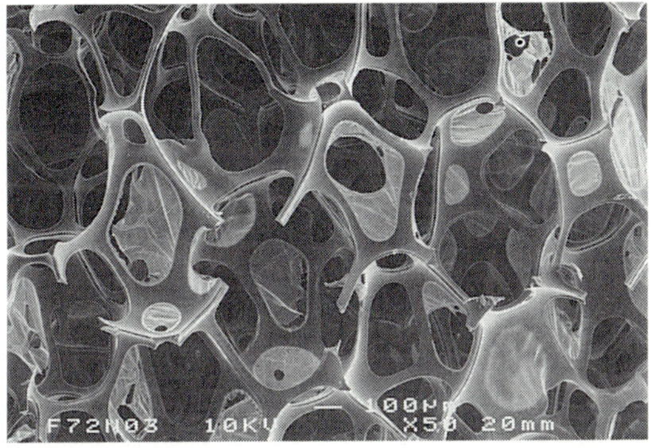

Figure 3

SEM micrographs of (a) Allevyn and (b) a competitor product (both are shown at a 50 × magnification)

The ability of a dressing to relieve pressure is also important. Pressure is defined as the force per unit area and a dressing must spread the load around the limb to reduce the pressure. The compressive properties of a foam relate to the pressure-relieving ability of the dressing in which it is incorporated.

The relationship between cell structure and mechanical properties has been well-studied(5). The load deflection curve for a foam in compression (Figure 4) shows an initial linear region (the slope of which is the initial modulus of the material) followed by a plateau and finally a rapid rise in load. The modulus can be related to the foam density — hence the cell dimensions — and is due to elastic bending of the cell edges. The plateau is caused by the buckling of the cell edges and the final rise in load is due to densification, ie compression of the now squashed cell edges. The important point in the graph as far as pressure reduction is concerned is the buckling point; above this the material will collapse and provide no further

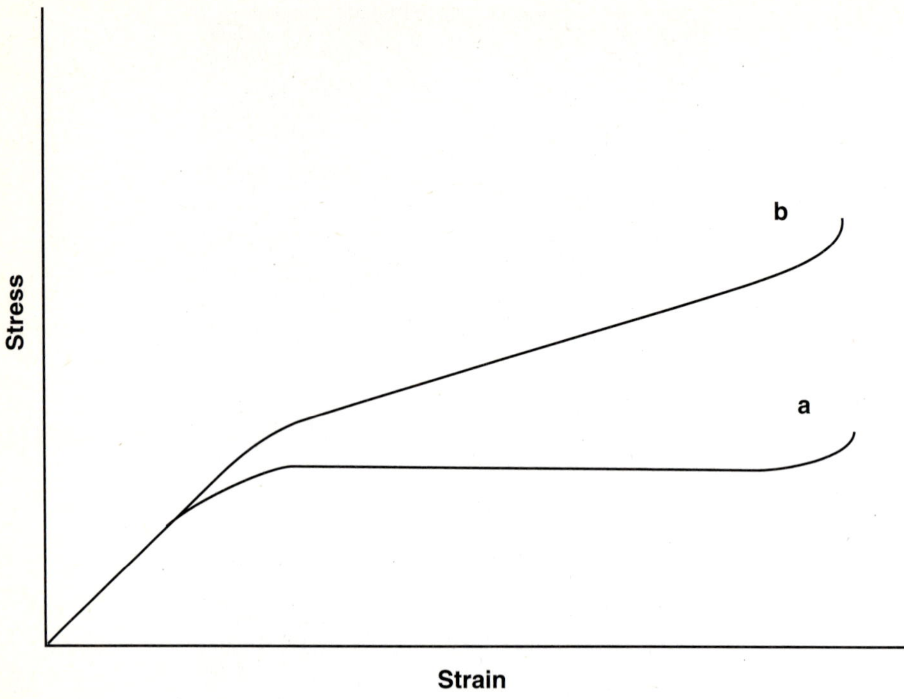

Figure 4

Ideal stress–strain curves for (a) a foam with uniform cell size and (b) a foam with a distribution of cell sizes

pressure relief. The compressive properties of a foam can therefore be improved by having a range of cells that buckle at different loads allowing the material to provide pressure relief over a much larger range of loads. A stress–strain curve for such a material is shown in Figure 4.

The compressive properties of the two dressings tested were measured (Figure 5) and the results showed that the Allevyn product has a higher initial buckling point and no horizontal plateau. Therefore, we would expect the Allevyn structure to contain both small cells and a range of cell sizes. In contrast, the competitor product has a low initial buckling point and an almost horizontal plateau, suggesting that it contains larger cells than are found in Allevyn and that the cells are uniform in size (Figure 4).

Conclusions

The rate of absorbency, fluid-retention and pressure-relieving properties of a cellular wound dressing are all affected by the structure of the cells within it. By understanding and

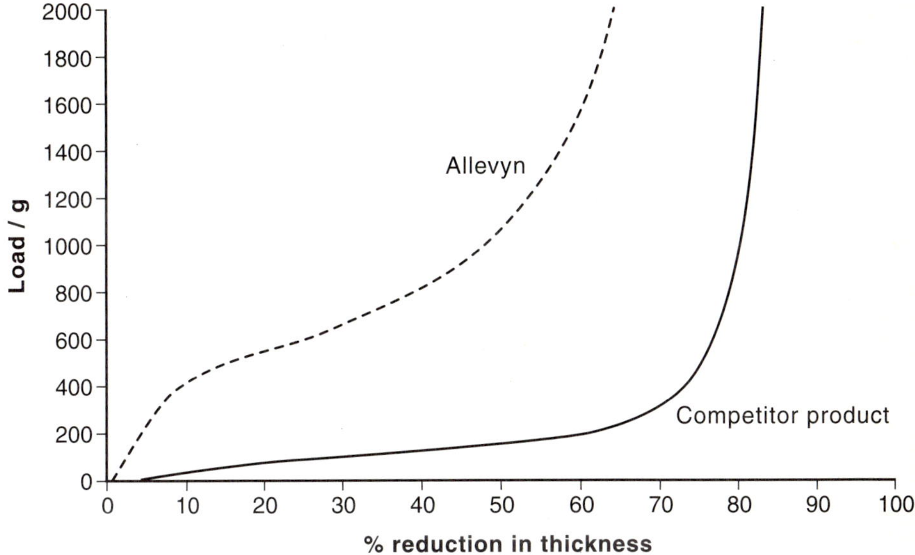

Figure 5

Measured load–compression curves for Allevyn and the competitor product

controlling the cell structure, a dressing can be designed with an optimal combination of properties.

References

1 Chatterjee PK. *Absorbency*. New York: Elsevier, 1985: 145.

2 Farrar D. *Internal Smith & Nephew report*, 1990.

3 Hagen G. Annalen der Physik und Chemie 1839; **46**: 423–42.

4 Poiseuille JL. *Comptes Rendus Acad Sci Paris* 1840; **11**: 961–1041.

5 Gibson LJ, Ashby MF. *Cellular solids — structure and properties*. New York: Pergamon Press, 1988.

Allevyn, an exudate manager: clinical experience

E RICCI, R CASSINO

DEPARTMENT OF VULNOLOGY,
NEW S. PAUL CLINIC, TURIN

Allevyn (Smith & Nephew) is a polyurethane foam dressing with a hydrocellular structure. It can be classified as a semipermeable dressing, like polyurethane films. Its main properties are to absorb exudate, maintain a moist environment and avoid maceration. The variety of sizes available means that it can be used to dress wounds of any shape or depth.

All chronic wounds must be viewed equally in terms of local treatment. The different aetiologies can influence choices about general treatment, but not about dressings. There are three different kinds of intervention in wound management:

- aetiopathogenetic therapy (directed at causation)
- therapy directed at the general host response (eg nutritional deficiency)
- local therapy (eg the dressing).

The first intervention is always different and dependent on the aetiology of the wound; the second is always the same and always necessary; the third, the dressing, is not related to aetiology, rather to the tissue of the wound. Ulcers caused by neoplastic and immune system diseases are the only exceptions.

Study aim

In any wound there are several features that can influence the choice of dressing: the type of wound, the type of tissue and the quantity of exudate. Allevyn, because of its absorptive properties, is indicated for all wound and tissue types. The aim of the present study was to

EVIDENCE-BASED WOUNDCARE, EDITED BY A SUGGETT, G CHERRY, R MANI, W EAGLSTEIN, 1998.
INTERNATIONAL CONGRESS AND SYMPOSIUM SERIES NO 227 PUBLISHED BY THE ROYAL SOCIETY OF MEDICINE PRESS LIMITED

evaluate the performance of Allevyn as both a primary and a secondary dressing, with particular regard to exudate control, wear time, healing rate and patient comfort.

Materials and methods

Allevyn was used to treat 54 patients with chronic wounds (66 lesions) of different aetiologies. Patients who displayed some or all of the following were excluded: clinical evidence of local infection; treatment with chemotherapeutic drugs; diseases of the immune system. Necrotic and sloughy lesions were treated as one group because the dressing used is the same in both; eschars were surgically debrided, removing the necrotic tissue at about 1 cm from the edge. All wounds were dressed after disinfection with normal saline solution. Dressings were changed every 72 hours when Allevyn was used as a secondary dressing. Dressings were changed in the event of detachment, leakage or saturation when Allevyn was used as a primary dressing. The size and shape of the dressings were chosen according to wound shape, avoiding the use of Allevyn Adhesive when perilesional skin was macerated.

Mean wear time was evaluated at the end of treatment; healing time was evaluated at complete debridement in the case of necrotic lesions and at healing in the case of granulating wounds. Maceration of perilesional skin was considered when evaluating exudate management and the following scores applied: 0 = normal skin; 1 = maceration (no skin lesion); 2 = epidermal lesion; 3 = dermal lesion. In cases of maceration, the interval of dressing change was reduced and data collected. Leakage was not considered. Comfort was evaluated during dressing change, with patients clarifying comfort as either good, satisfactory or poor.

Table 1 *Results according to aetiology; times in days*

Aetiology	Number	Wear time	Healing time	Debriding time
Pressure sores	36	3.7	48.6	10.1
Venous ulcers	20	5.6	56.3	7
Arterial venous ulcers	6	3.2	79.2	15.2
Diabetic foot ulcers	4	4.1	171.5	18
Total	66	4.3	88.9	11.6

Table 2 *Granulating wound; Allevyn employed as a primary dressing*

		Maceration score				
Exudate	Number	0	1	2	3	Wear time
Low	22	21	1	—	—	6.6
Medium	22	18	4	—	—	3.4
Heavy	6	0	2	3	1	1.9
Total	50	39	7	3	1	

0=normal skin; 1=maceration (no skin lesion); 2=epidermal lesion; 3=dermal lesion

Table 3 *Necrotic wound; Allevyn employed as a secondary dressing*

		Maceration score			
Exudate	Number	0	1	2	3
Low	4	4	—	—	—
Medium	8	4	2	1	1
Heavy	4	2	1	—	1
Total	16	10	3	1	2

0=normal skin; 1=maceration (no skin lesion); 2=epidermal lesion; 3=dermal lesion

Results

Every wound in the study was considered and evaluated. Table 1 shows the overall results on wear time, healing time and debriding time, according to aetiology. Maceration was important in this study in terms of the evaluation of exudate management. The score assessing exudate level is shown in granulating ulcers (Table 2) and necrotic ulcers (Table 3). Maceration was found in 24.2% of treated ulcers but resolution required more than seven days in only three cases (4.5%) and the dressing never had to be changed. Comfort was good in 77.3% of cases, satisfactory in 15.2% and poor in 7.5%. No adverse reactions and no clinical evidence of infection were reported.

Discussion

Polyurethane foam can clearly work both as a primary and secondary dressing in the management of exudate. According to this study, Allevyn can be considered a safe dressing because no complications, adverse reactions or infections were reported. Maceration is very common in heavily exuding wounds, but only one case (2%) of maceration was recorded when Allevyn was used as a primary dressing, and two cases (12.5%) when it was used as a secondary dressing. The authors concluded that such maceration was due to too long an interval between dressing changes.

Session 3
EVIDENCE ON QUALITY OF LIFE

A review of the impact of dressings on quality of life

PC BAULING

205 MEDFORUM, PRETORIA, SOUTH AFRICA

The patient's perspective

Quality of life assessment as a tool in health care delivery was defined by Fallowfield in 1990 as a combination of four primary domains: psychological, social, occupational and physical[1]. Clinicians might find it surprising that the psychological domain is listed first. A review of the literature reinforces the belief that every patient with acute or chronic wounds should be asked what impact the injury has had on his or her life. A management plan should then be worked out in consultation with the patient, including a discussion on limitations and shortcomings.

It is important to be aware of the individual needs of every patient, to coordinate these with knowledge of the available dressings for a particular injury and to work out a plan of action unique to the patient's needs and the available resources. This plan of action constitutes an evidence-based approach to a quality of life management plan. Its application assumes total commitment by well-informed and fully-resourced doctors, nurses and patients although, unfortunately, this is not always the case.

It is important to understand the impact of the wound on the individual's quality of life before reviewing the impact of dressings. A significant body of information has been produced over the past five to ten years on quality of life impairment, focusing mainly on chronic wounds[2–4]. It is surprising to discover from current literature that pain, in particular in venous ulcer disease, is excruciating and significant and that in standard textbooks it is not often mentioned[5]. Other important patient complaints, of which clinicians are not always aware,

EVIDENCE-BASED WOUNDCARE, EDITED BY A SUGGETT, G CHERRY, R MANI, W EAGLSTEIN, 1998.
INTERNATIONAL CONGRESS AND SYMPOSIUM SERIES NO 227 PUBLISHED BY THE ROYAL SOCIETY OF MEDICINE PRESS LIMITED

include loss of both sleep and mobility. Patients also complain that health care professionals do not listen to them and that they have a sense of helplessness and hopelessness. Patient quotes include: 'I'm going off my head'; 'I had to close my business'; 'I never go on holiday, cannot bath'[3].

It should be clear from this list of quality of life impairments that clinicians sometimes have a very poor understanding of patients' concerns. Although no amount of encouragement, explanation and discussion on the proposed strategy for care and treatment of the wound can ever be wasted on a patient, all too often the patient's needs are completely ignored in the consideration of management options.

Dressing impact on quality of life: acute injury/burns

In modern times a dressing may be defined as any material or covering applied to a patient—either locally or systemically—that aims to have a positive influence on wound healing and quality of life, ie systemic administration of tissue growth factors, cadaver skin, xenogeneic skin etc. For example, a general statement that can be supported by the evidence-based approach is that rapid surgical skin coverage in burn injuries has a tremendous impact on quality of life, both in partial- and full-thickness burns. It should be remembered that skin grafts immediately remove all wound pain in a grafted area[6–8]. The donor site could and should also be pain-free within a period of three to ten days, which could vastly improve quality of life. The management of donor sites by burn surgeons represents a true test of their evidence-based approach and quality of life goals. It is important to heal the donor site quickly as it is the main source of pain in most burn patients.

Several authors have reviewed studies on moist wound healing in partial-thickness burns and these reports clearly show an excellent improvement in quality of life[9,10]. A database of evidence shows that pig skin, cadaver skin, Granuflex (Duoderm) and Omiderm are some of the products that accelerate the re-epithelialization of partial thickness burns, compared with daily silver sulphadiazine dressings. Patients are additionally spared the painful and traumatizing experience of daily dressing changes.

Dressing impact on quality of life: chronic wounds

Using quality of life standards, what can be considered the most advanced management for chronic wounds? Some products—such as Granuflex (Duoderm), Omiderm, hydrofibres and compression bandaging—certainly have some evidence to support their use in chronic wounds, but other products — such as vacuum-assisted healing, growth factors and others — need further evaluation before clear evidence is produced of an associated improvement in quality of life. Although it seems that all of the modern modalities have brought about significant quality of life improvement, in terms of randomized controlled trials there is no substantial body of evidence to prove that this is the case. Many studies exist, but most fail on study design defects (insufficient numbers or lack of control of other variables)[11,12]. Despite the lack of evidence, these products have made an impact and led to the drawing up of clinical guidelines based on the moist wound healing concept.

It is important to appreciate that not all chronic wounds are the same and manageable with one universal dressing. Most dressing products have only marginal advantages over one another. Judgement, experience and product knowledge are all essential to a successful quality of life improvement approach. There are however some cautions: not all hydrocolloids are identical in terms of pH management, gas exchange, pectin content, fibroblast toxicity, glue properties and duration of action; similarly not all polyurethane films are the same.

Using quality of life as the standard, the optimal dressing protocol must first alleviate pain so that the patient can function uninhibited during the day and sleep at night. It must also achieve significant reintegration of the patient on a psychological, social, functional and economic level. An ideal dressing would speed up healing, reduce or abolish odour and exudate, allow painless application and removal, have a long wear time, achieve excellent patient compliance and be cost-effective. Issues of importance to patients, after pain relief, include:

- adequate mobility
- unembarrassing and preferably invisible dressing
- ability to continue working and socializing
- minimal interference with bathing and sexual activity.

Patients do not want to be hospitalized, confined to bed or have their legs elevated.

Conclusion

Chronic wound care has greatly improved since the introduction of ambulatory home care, a variety of modern dressings, and — where there are clear and unequivocal signs of local or systemic infection — use of antimicrobial therapy. There is no universal dressing: the clinician must use the right dressing at the right time to improve a patient's quality of life. To heal a wound is not difficult, but to heal a wound in a scientific and humane way is an art.

References

1 Fallowfield L. *The quality of life: the missing dimension in health care.* London: Souvenir, 1990: 3–16.

2 Walshe C. Living with a leg ulcer: a descriptive study of patients' experience. *J Adv Nursing* 1995; **22**: 1092–100.

3 Charles H. The impact of leg ulcers on patients' quality of life. *Professional Nurse* 1995; **10**: 571–4.

4 Nelissen E, Evers G, Degreef H, Flour M. Scoring discomfort caused by chronic wounds and wound care: can we improve our treatment protocols? In: Leaper DJ, Dealey C, Cherry GW, *et al*, eds. *Proceedings of the sixth European Conference on Advances in Wound Management.* London: Macmillan Magazines Ltd, 1990: 60.

5 Morris PJ, Malt RA, eds. *Oxford Textbook of Surgery on Compact Disc.* Oxford University Press & AND Electronic Publishing, 1995: 1229.

6 Monafo WW. Then and now: 50 years of burn treatment. *Burns* 1992; **18**(suppl): S7–S10.

7 Janzekowic Z. A new concept in early excision and immediate grafting of burns. *J Trauma* 1970; **10**: 1103–8.

8 Heimbach DM. Early burn excision and grating. *Surg Clin North Am* 1987; **67**: 93–107.

9 Hickerson WL, Kealey GP, Smith DJ Jr, Thomson PD. A prospective comparison of a new synthetic donor site dressing versus an impregnated gauze dressing. *J Burn Care & Rehab* 1994; **15**: 359–63.

10 Hermans MHE. Treatment of burns with occlusive dressings: some pathophysiologic and quality of life aspects. Burns 1992; **18**(suppl): S515–18.

11 Bolton L, Faltu A. Topical agents and wound healing clinics. *Dermatology* 1994; **12**: 95–120, 150.

12 Ter Riet G, Kessels AGH, Knipschild P. Keynote address: Wound healing—problems in the conduct of a randomized trial. In: Leaper DJ, Dealey C, Cherry GW, *et al*, eds. *Proceedings of the sixth European Conference on Advances in Wound Management.* London: Macmillan Magazines Ltd, 1990: 121–4.

Quality of life assessment in wound management

P PRICE

WOUND HEALING RESEARCH UNIT, UNIVERSITY OF WALES COLLEGE OF MEDICINE, CARDIFF, UK

Health-related quality of life (HRQOL) is a concept that has attracted increasing attention over the past 10 years. The research focus has been on the development of ways of defining and measuring the concept so that it can be used in three key areas:

- research and audit
- clinical management
- policy setting.

In areas such as oncology, work on HRQOL has already been undertaken for a number of years. The result is a substantial body of evidence supporting the idea that an individual's attitude towards their condition (and the initial level of HRQOL) can impact on health outcomes.

Definitions have been put forward to aid the understanding of the concept of HRQOL; these have ranged from the very broad, reflecting the difference between current and desired status[1], to a listing of specific domains to be measured[2]. Currently there is some consensus[3] that the concept should focus on investigating the impact of a disease or disorder on everyday living in key areas such as physical functioning, social functioning and wellbeing. The range of decisions that researchers and clinicians have to face when deciding to use a HRQOL measure is outlined below.

A number of generic tools (eg SF-36) have been developed to compare the impact of a number of chronic conditions on everyday living. These assess different health states, then compare the results to a table of norms to determine the differences.

EVIDENCE-BASED WOUNDCARE, EDITED BY A SUGGETT, G CHERRY, R MANI, W EAGLSTEIN, 1998.
INTERNATIONAL CONGRESS AND SYMPOSIUM SERIES NO 227 PUBLISHED BY THE ROYAL SOCIETY OF MEDICINE PRESS LIMITED

Condition-specific measures are, in contrast, designed to be sensitive to the impact of a particular disorder or disease and are more likely to be sensitive to minor changes in overall health state, which represent significant clinical differences. A substantial amount of time is required to develop a new condition-specific tool, as sound psychometric properties must be established in order to ensure its validity, reliability, sensitivity and discriminatory powers[4].

A choice must also be made between the use of a profile or index approach to measurement. Profiles are often preferred in the clinical or research setting, since they provide information on a range of aspects of everyday living. However, those working in the health policy or health economics environment tend to prefer tools that result in a single index, particularly when sophisticated cost analyses are performed.

It should be noted that many of these methods are relatively new and at various stages of development.

HRQOL and chronic wounds

The work that has been completed in relation to HRQOL and chronic wounds falls into three categories: qualitative approaches, use of generic HRQOL measures and the development of disease-specific HRQOL measures.

The following is not a complete review of the literature, but gives a sound indication of the work completed to date.

Qualitative approaches

In 1994 Phillips *et al* outlined the results of standardized personal interviews with 62 patients[5]. These patients reported that the most difficult aspects of living with a chronic wound were pain and the impact on mobility; younger patients reported concern about the financial impact on their lives. A majority (68%) reported a negative psychological impact, including depression and anxiety and 58% found that caring for their wound was 'burdensome'.

In 1995 Walshe[6] reported the results of a small study (n=13) using in-depth interviews analysed using phenomenography. Again pain and impact on mobility were seen as the major difficulties.

Generic measures

Generic measures of HRQOL have been designed to look at the impact of any given disorder on everyday living, and compare any group of patients with age- and sex-matched norms established for the health population. These tools allow for comparisons across a variety of disorders and diseases.

In 1993 Lindholm published the results of a study of 125 patients (51 men, 74 women) from Sweden who completed the Nottingham Health Profile[7]. The results revealed gender differences indicating that the impact on men may be greater than that on women, with respect to pain, emotional reaction, social isolation and physical mobility.

In 1996 Price and Harding conducted a study using the SF-36, adopted by the WHO as the 'gold standard' of generic measures[8]. This study of 63 patients (37 women) showed that on seven of the eight subscales, patients with chronic wounds rated themselves as significantly poorer than age-matched norms. Gender differences in this study indicated that the impact on women might be greater; the contrast with Lindholm's study may be due to differences in sampling, tool used, or methods of statistical analysis. This study also showed that patients with a wound >24 months old reported less pain and better general health, possibly as a result of adaptation to the condition. However, when this patient group was followed up four months later, the SF-36 did not discriminate between healed and unhealed wounds.

Disease-specific measures

While disease-specific measures have been developed for chronic wounds, two tools have been developed for related areas — the Freiburg Quality of Life Assessment[9] and The Chronic Lower Limb Venous Insufficiency Scale[10].

In 1994 Franks *et al* reported on a study of 168 patients at two time points[11]. Using The Symptoms Rating Test and interviews, Franks investigated the impact of community care on patients with chronic wounds. The results indicate a reduction in mean scores for anxiety, depression and hostility over time (although the analysis did not compare those who healed with those who did not). Patients also reported a significant reduction in pain and 'bother' associated with wound care and an increase in general health affecting leisure activities.

The development of a new tool for patients with chronic wounds has been outlined by Hyland, Ley and Thompson (1994)[12]. This study shows the progress of the tool from initial interviews with focus groups (*n*=6), through a pilot study (*n*=33) and then a main study (*n*=50) outlining the results of Factor Analysis which revealed that one factor underlies the 29-item questionnaire, ie the scale items can be added together to give one score. This study reports that the primary effects of the wound are pain, sleep disturbance and impaired mobility.

As part of the development work of a new disease-specific tool — The Cardiff Wound Impact Schedule — Price *et al*[13] produced a checklist of different causes of stress to investigate the difficulties patients experience when living with a chronic wound. This study included patients with chronic leg ulceration as well as diabetic foot ulceration, but there were no significant differences between the groups for any of the results. Patients were asked to rate items at two time points, four months apart, to see if the patient perceptions changed with time. Many of the items reported as stressful at time point 1 were still thought to be stressful at time point 2 (eg fear of damaging the wound). Certain items, not considered very stressful at time point 1 were rated much higher at time point 2 (eg discomfort of bandaging, feeling dirty). This study served to remind us that patient's views are not necessarily static and may change over time.

Use in clinical trials

Unlike other chronic conditions, there are very few clinical trials in woundcare that have included a HRQOL measure. However, Franks *et al* in 1995[14] published a paper that compared single- and multi-layer bandaging in patients with chronic venous ulceration. This was a large study of 200 patients who were asked to complete the Nottingham Health Profile. All scores improved over a 24-week period and the four-layer bandaging system was associated with greater improvement in energy and mobility.

An overview of work to date

The work in this area is relatively new; a range of methodologies and measures are being applied in order to ascertain which are the most appropriate in this patient population. Many of the studies are cross-sectional in design and descriptive in nature, indicating that there is still a large amount of basic theoretical and empirical work yet to be completed. The disease-specific tools are also relatively new and it will still be some time before they are used as part of routine care.

The term 'quality of life' is becoming overused, increasing the risk of it being used either inappropriately or indiscriminately[15]. This could lead to disenchantment with the term by health professionals, patients, and researchers, but the work is important and this should not be allowed to happen.

What is the value of HRQOL?

Reasons for continuing work in this area can be grouped under four main headings:

Clinical

Although the term HRQOL is relatively new, it is quite clear that health professionals are—and have been for some time—intuitively taking account of HRQOL issues when making clinical decisions. Further work will help us to formalize some of these decisions and assist clinicians in working within the framework of evidence-based medicine. HRQOL data may be particularly relevant when expensive or hazardous options need to be considered.

Research

Over the past 50 years there has been a growing awareness that the focus of health care is shifting away from acute conditions towards chronic conditions, in which perfect health or complete healing may not be a realistic option. In such cases, HRQOL data may prove to be a useful additional research outcome measure.

Audit

HRQOL data may be extremely useful within audit, demonstrating effectiveness and as a means of measuring change. If the clinical audit aim is to identify and remedy deficiencies in health care provision, HRQOL will allow us a patient-based view of the service and treatment provided.

Financial

In an economic climate in which there are finite resources but unlimited demand, HRQOL could help provide a framework for important policy decisions on expenditure. There is, as yet, no 'gold standard' measure of cost-effectiveness and, in the development of appropriate formulae, the 'human' cost will need to be considered. Work on utility analysis has attempted to find a measure which aggregates 'quantity' and 'quality' of life into a single index.

Conclusion

There has been an explosion of interest in HRQOL over the past 10 years and this has resulted in researchers attempting to address difficult conceptual questions about the meaning of 'quality' in everyday life. The development of a range of generic and condition-specific tools which allow us to investigate HRQOL within a scientific framework has resulted but there is still work to be done.

Since the issues relating to HRQOL can be quite emotive, surely we should attempt to deal with patients in such a way that their quality of life is one of our main priorities? The question in a tight economic climate is: Are we prepared to ensure that such measures are part of a total package of health care?

References

1 Calman KC. Quality of life in cancer patients—an hypothesis. *J Med Ethics* 1984, **10**: 124–7.

2 Fallowfield L. *Quality of life: the missing dimension in health care*. London: Souvenir, 1990.

3 Patrick DL, Erickson P. Assessing health-related quality of life for clinical decision-making. In: Walker SR, Rosser RM, eds. *Quality of life assessment: key issues for the 1990s*. London: Kluwer Academic Publishers, 1993: 11–63.

4 Price PE, Harding KG. Defining quality of life. *J Wound Care* 1993; **2**(5): 304–6.

5 Phillips T, Stanton B, Provan A, Lew R. A study of the impact of leg ulcers on quality of life: financial, social and psychologic implications. *J Am Acad Dermatol* 1994; **31**: 49–55.

6 Walshe C. Living with a venous leg ulcer: a descriptive study of patients' experiences. *J Advanced Nursing* 1995; **22**: 1092–100.

7 Lindholm C, Bjellerup M, Christensen OB, Zederfeldt B. Quality of life in chronic leg ulcer patients: an assessment according to the Nottingham Health Profile. *Acta Derm Venereol (Stockh)* 1993; **73**: 440–3.

8 Price P, Harding K. Measuring health-related quality of life in patients with chronic leg ulcers. *Wounds* 1996; **8**(3): 91–4.

9 Augustin M, Dieterle W, Zschocke I, *et al.* Development and validation of a disease-specific questionnaire on the quality of life from patients with chronic venous insufficiency. *Fourth annual conference, International Society of Quality of Life Research*. Vienna, 1997.

10 Launois R, Reboul-Marty J, Henry B. Construction and validation of a quality of life questionnaire in chronic lower limb insufficiency (CIVIQ). *Quality of Life Research* 1996; **5**(6): 539–54.

11 Franks PJ, Moffatt CJ, Connolly M, *et al.* Community leg ulcer clinics: effects on quality of life. *Phlebology* 1994; **9**: 83–6.

12 Hyland ME, Ley A, Thompson B. Quality of life in leg ulcer patients: questionnaire and preliminary findings. *J Wound Care* 1994; **3**(6): 294–8.

13 Price PE, Keeling D, Harding KG. Changes in chronic wound related stressors over a four month period. *Symposium on Advanced Wound Care & Medical Research Forum on Wound Repair*. New Orleans, 1997.

14 Franks PJ, Bosanquet N, Brown D, *et al.* Received health in randomised trials of single and multi-layer bandaging for chronic venous ulceration. *Phlebology* 1995; **1**(suppl): 17–19.

15 Fairclough D. Quality of life in cancer clinical trials: the clinical perspective. *Fourth annual conference of International Society of Quality of Life*. Vienna, 1997.

A multicentre pilot study to investigate the physical performance of a novel Allevyn Adhesive dressing

M BENBOW

MID-CHESHIRE HOSPITALS TRUST, LEIGHTON HOSPITAL, CREWE, CHESHIRE, UK

Allevyn Adhesive dressings (Smith & Nephew) were launched in 1987. Since then they have been successfully used to treat a variety of wounds including leg ulcers, diabetic foot ulcers and skin graft donor sites[1–5]. Comparative clinical studies have shown that the dressings encourage healing, relieve pain and provide a cost-effective treatment[1,2,6].

The purpose of this study was to evaluate the performance of a new Allevyn Adhesive dressing through the assessment of ease of use, absorbency and durability and to compare its performance with that of a hydrocolloid dressing. The collaborating centres were Cardiff, Doncaster (two sites), Darlington and Crewe.

Methods

This study chose a randomized, prospective comparison of Allevyn Adhesive dressings and Granuflex hydrocolloid dressings. Patients had stage 2 or 3 pressure sores, with a wound size $\leqslant 11$ cm and no signs of clinical infection. On entry, a brief history was obtained from each patient and their wound examined and assessed. A further assessment of the selected wound was made when the patient was discharged. Patients were discharged when their wound healed, after 30 days, or until they were withdrawn from the study, whichever occurred first.

EVIDENCE-BASED WOUNDCARE, EDITED BY A SUGGETT, G CHERRY, R MANI, W EAGLSTEIN, 1998.
INTERNATIONAL CONGRESS AND SYMPOSIUM SERIES NO 227 PUBLISHED BY THE ROYAL SOCIETY OF MEDICINE PRESS LIMITED

Statistical methods

Data were entered, verified, validated and analysed using a statistical analysis system (SAS). All tests were two-sided and the 5% level considered 'significant' in accordance with usual practice. All parameters assessed were analysed using the Mann–Whitney test, except for the mean dressing wear time which was analysed using the Student's *t* test.

Results

Of the patients recruited, 40/61 were withdrawn. The main reasons for this were death or discharge before wounds healed. None of the deaths was considered to be dressing-related. Sometimes a combination of factors was involved in withdrawal. Five patients in the Allevyn group were discharged home or transferred to nursing homes before their wounds healed or before they had completed the study period. The high withdrawal rate is a problem experienced when conducting trials involving patients with pressure sores.

The statistical analysis involved 60 patients. The groups were well-balanced for age, sex, and stage and site of pressure sore (Table 1). Most sores were identified as stage 2 and situated either on the heels or sacrum. Sores dressed with Granuflex were slightly larger than those dressed with Allevyn Adhesive.

Table 1 *Patient data*

	Allevyn Adhesive	Granuflex
Number of patients	29	31
Age (median)	73 years	74 years
Sex		
Male	12 (41%)	15 (48%)
Female	17 (59%)	16 (52%)
Sore location		
Sacrum	18 (62%)	13 (42%)
Trochanter	1 (3%)	1 (3%)
Heel	5 (17%)	11 (35%)
Other	5 (17%)	6 (19%)
Stage of sore		
2	23 (79%)	22 (71%)
3	6 (21%)	9 (29%)

Twelve of the wounds healed during the trial; seven in the Allevyn group and five in the Granuflex group. A further nine patients completed the study with unhealed wounds at 30 days (five in the Allevyn group and four in the Granuflex group). Eighteen subjects were withdrawn in the Allevyn group and 22 in the Granuflex group. There was only one dressing-related adverse incident in the Allevyn group, in the form of a localized skin rash.

Most of the dressings were rated 'easy to apply'. Allevyn Adhesive was rated as significantly better at conforming to body contours. The absorbency of Allevyn Adhesive was reported to be superior to Granuflex (Figure 1). Dressing absorbency was rated as 'good' in 81% of Allevyn dressings, compared with 26% of Granuflex dressings. In the Allevyn group there was soiling of bedclothes in 4% of cases compared with 25% in the Granuflex group. The mean wear times for the two dressings were not significantly different (3.8 days in the Allevyn group and 3.2 days in the Granuflex group).

Allevyn Adhesive dressing was significantly easier to remove than Granuflex (Figure 2). There were no reports of Allevyn causing wound damage but Granuflex was reported as causing

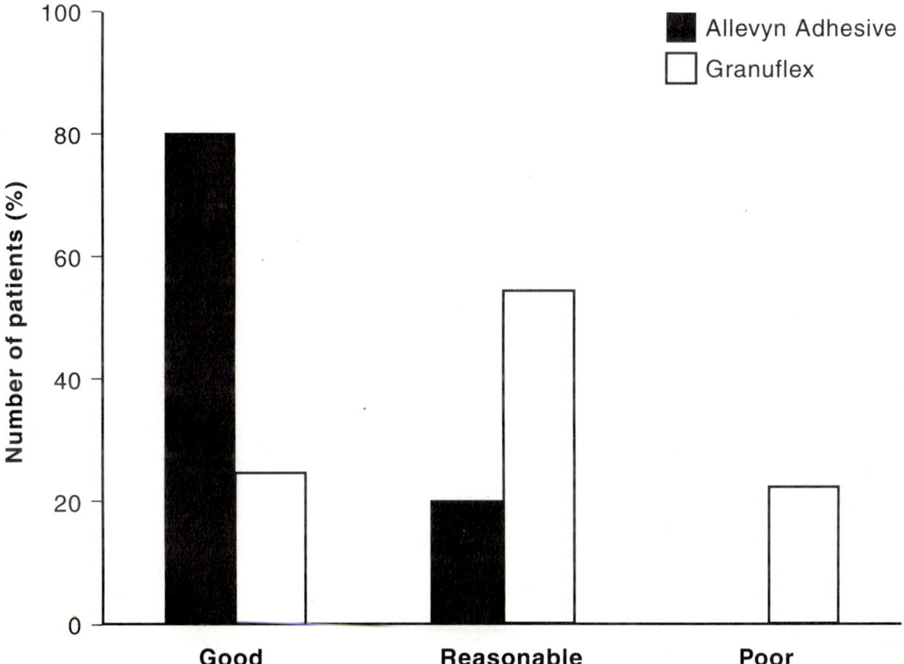

Figure 1

Dressing absorbency

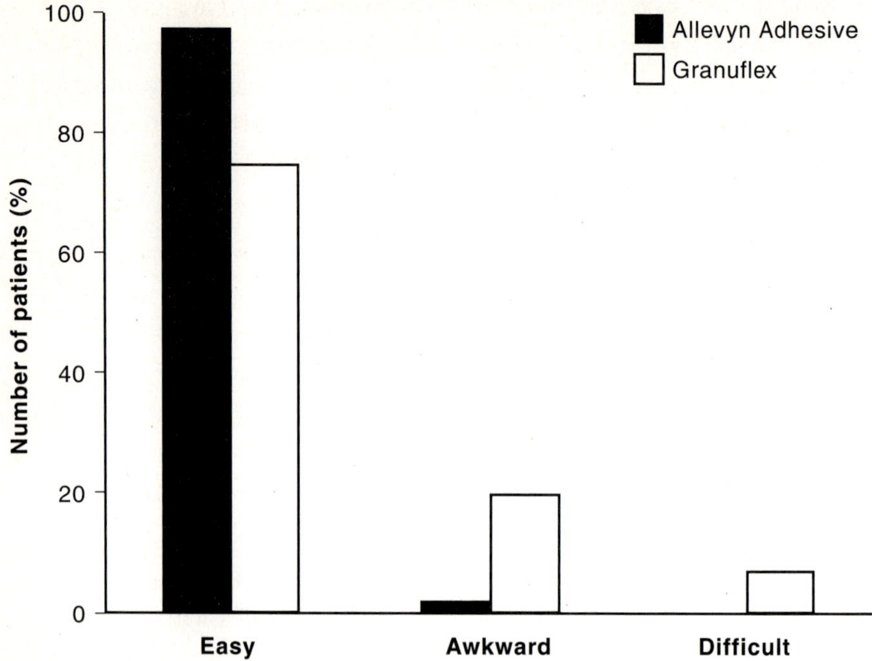

Figure 2
Ease of dressing removal

damage in 3% of cases. Damage to surrounding skin was reported in 2% of Allevyn cases and 7% of Granuflex cases.

Conclusion

The study results indicate that the absorbency of Allevyn is superior to that of Granuflex; this is supported by fewer reports of soiling of clothes and bedclothes in the Allevyn group. Mean wear times in both groups were similar. Although 'loss of adhesion' was the most common reason for changing dressings, it is likely that this reflects the instruction to investigators — that they should leave dressings for as long as possible — rather than poor performance of the adhesive.

References

1 Callam MJ, Harper DR, Dale JJ, *et al.* Lothian and Forth Valley leg ulcer healing trial, part 2. Knitted viscose dressing versus a hydrocellular dressing in the treatment of chronic leg ulceration. *Phlebology* 1992; **7**: 142–5.

2 Zuccarelli F. A study to evaluate and compare the performance of a hydrocellular dressing with a hydrocolloid dressing in the treatment of venous leg ulcers. In: *Proceedings of the second European conference on advances in wound management.* London: Macmillan Magazines Ltd, 1993.

3 Foster AVM, Greenhill MT, Edmonds E. Comparing two dressings in the treatment of diabetic foot ulcers. *J Wound Care* 1994; **3**(5): 224–8.

4 Baker NR, Creevy J. A randomised comparative pilot study to evaluate Allevyn hydrocellular dressings and Sorbsan calcium alginate dressings in the treatment of diabetic foot ulcers. In: *Proceedings of the third European conference on advances in wound management.* London: Macmillan Magazines Ltd, 1994.

5 Hankins PD, Limitone E, Weber RS. A randomised study comparing wound coverage of split thickness skin graft donor sites. A poster presented at: *The fifth Symposium on Advanced Wound Care*. New Orleans, 1992.

6 Bale S, Banks B, Orpin J, Harding KG. Setting standards for cost-effectiveness studies: a trial of Allevyn hydrocellular dressing and a hydrocolloid dressing. In: *Proceedings of the fourth European conference on advances in wound management.* London: Macmillan Magazines Ltd, 1995.

Session 4

EVIDENCE IN LEG ULCER THERAPY

A comparative study of four-layer and single-layer elastic bandages in limb oedema

G SIBBALD

UNIVERSITY OF TORONTO, ONTARIO, CANADA

Single-layer elastic bandaging is the most common type of compression used in Canada. This single-centre, prospective, randomized, parallel group study compared four-layer compression bandaging with single-layer elastic bandaging in an attempt to correlate the reduction of limb oedema in patients suffering from chronic venous insufficiency with the healing of leg ulceration. The aim was to provide evidence to support the more widespread introduction of four-layer bandaging into Canadian clinical practice.

Materials and methods

Forty-three patients with venous leg ulcers and an ankle brachial pressure index >0.8 entered the study. The major exclusion criteria were other dermatological disorders that might cause problems with bandaging, pentoxifylline or Trental therapy, use of agents that interfere with healing (such as immunosuppressives or corticosteroids), malignancy, vasculitis or neurotrophic ulcers, pregnancy, or previous entry to the study. The study consisted of 65% women and 35% men, with a mean age of 65. Twenty-two patients were randomized to receive four-layer bandages and 21 elastic bandages. Baseline variables were balanced, but initial ulcer areas were slightly higher in the elastic bandage group. Oedema was measured using limb circumference measurements and water displacement of the limb after venous refilling.

EVIDENCE-BASED WOUNDCARE, EDITED BY A SUGGETT, G CHERRY, R MANI, W EAGLSTEIN, 1998.
INTERNATIONAL CONGRESS AND SYMPOSIUM SERIES NO 227 PUBLISHED BY THE ROYAL SOCIETY OF MEDICINE PRESS LIMITED

Results

The wounds of seven patients in the four-layer group (32%), and three patients in the elastic group (14%) healed in less than six weeks. Of the remaining patients, 13 of 14 in the four-layer and 15 of 18 in the elastic bandage groups finished the six-week study.

Statistically significant differences between the bandaging types were seen for foot circumference ($p<0.001$) and mid-calf circumference ($p=0.003$), using the Stepwise analysis of variance model. No statistically significant difference between the bandaging types was seen for limb volume ($p=0.59$, NS). The remaining measurements (ankle circumference and upper-calf circumference) were more reduced in the four-layer than in the elastic group, but the differences were not statistically significant ($p=0.55$ and $p=0.17$ NS respectively). There were no statistically significant differences seen for the main percentage change from baseline in ulcer area ($p=0.22$) or for the time to healing experienced by patients on the two bandaging regimes ($p=0.17$).

Conclusion

Four-layer bandaging provides good limb oedema control, particularly in terms of foot and mid-calf circumference reduction, compared to single-layer bandaging.

Evaluation of surface pH on venous leg ulcers under Allevyn dressings

M ROMANELLI, E SCHIPANI, A PIAGGESI, P BARACHINI

DEPARTMENT OF DERMATOLOGY AND DEPARTMENT OF METABOLIC DISEASES, UNIVERSITY OF PISA, ITALY

The surface pH of chronic wounds can differ according to the stage of healing. Prolonged chemical acidification of the wound surface has been shown to enhance the healing rate of venous leg ulcers(1) and the moist environment obtained under occlusive dressings greatly increases the healing rate of chronic wounds(2). Tsukada and colleagues(3), using pH measurement of pressure ulcers, were able to correlate different pH values to various stages of healing and to assess the epithelialization of a wound. In this study the surface pH of venous leg ulcers was measured at different intervals after the application of a hydrocellular dressing.

Patients and methods

We prospectively evaluated 23 patients (eight men, 15 women, mean age 64±8) attending our leg ulcer clinic as outpatients. They all presented with clinical and objective evidence of a chronic venous leg ulcer (ankle brachial pressure index >0.8), had at least 75% of the wound bed area covered with granulation tissue and were not on any systemic therapy. Ulcers were dressed with a hydrocellular foam, Allevyn Adhesive (Smith & Nephew) and the surface pH of the wound bed was measured with a flat glass pH electrode (pH C2441, Radiometer, Denmark) connected to a pH meter (PHM 82 standard pH meter, Radiometer, Denmark). The instrument was calibrated before each measurement, using standard pH solutions of 4 and 7.

EVIDENCE-BASED WOUNDCARE, EDITED BY A SUGGETT, G CHERRY, R MANI, W EAGLSTEIN, 1998.
INTERNATIONAL CONGRESS AND SYMPOSIUM SERIES NO 227 PUBLISHED BY THE ROYAL SOCIETY OF MEDICINE PRESS LIMITED

Measurements were taken at baseline, 48 hours and 72 hours. They were taken immediately after dressing removal and before applying any detergent, to avoid changes in wound-bed pH. The electrode was rested, without applying force, on the wound bed and three consecutive readings taken at the same site, with an interval of 2 minutes between each reading. The mean ±standard deviation (SD) was considered the effective pH value; normal skin proximal to the ulcer and under the dressing was used for a control measurement. Skin temperature was measured at the same time as pH measurement, with a non-contact infrared thermometer (Calex Raytek, ST2). The analysis of variance (Anova) test was used for statistical analysis and statistical significance defined as $p<0.05$.

Results

Surface pH measurements of the venous leg ulcers and control skin are shown in Figure 1. Baseline pH values of the wound bed (8.2±1.5) were significantly higher than those of normal skin (5.2±0.6) ($p<0.05$). When the dressing was removed at 48 hours, the wound was weakly acidic with a pH of 6.4±0.4. This acidic environment continued at dressing removal after 72 hours, with a pH of 6.2±0.2 (a value not significantly different to the 48 hour measurement at the same site). Control skin maintained its acidic environment from baseline to the end of the study with a mean pH of 5.4±0.5. There were no significant differences in skin temperature between the ulcer bed and normal skin at dressing removal during the study.

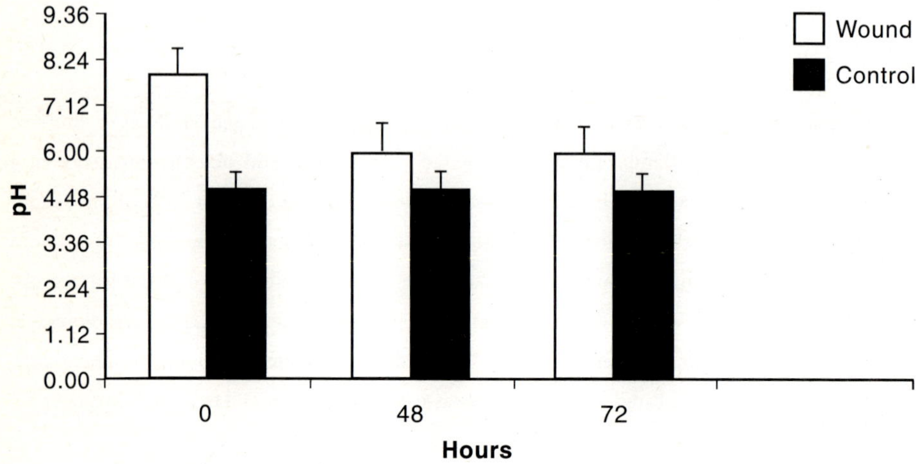

Figure 1

Surface pH of wound bed and normal skin at different intervals under a hydrocellular foam dressing

Discussion

This study demonstrated that a hydrocellular foam dressing was able to turn the pH of venous granulating leg ulcers from alkaline to acidic and to maintain this acidic environment up to dressing removal at 72 hours. The foam dressing used, because of its highly absorbent capacity, has the potential to be left in place on chronic wounds for an even longer period, avoiding frequent dressing changes.

The acidic pH found under synthetic dressings has been shown to inhibit bacterial growth and to promote fibroblast proliferation in chronic wounds[4]. The mechanism underlying these events is unclear, but seems related to the increase in oxygen release which causes a shift to the right in the haemoglobin–oxyhaemoglobin dissociation curve[5]. Measurement of surface pH is a non-invasive technique which has been used in the past to evaluate the barrier properties of the stratum corneum after application of a synthetic detergent[6], to predict skin graft survival[7], and to study the relationship between change in skin surface pH and the development of skin irritation[8].

In this study we found pH measurement of the wound bed a rapid, easy and reproducible method.

References

1 Wilson IAI, Henry M, Quill RD, *et al.* The pH of varicose ulcer surfaces and its relationship to healing. *VASA* 1979; **8**: 339–42.

2 Ryan TJ. Wound dressing. *Dermatol Clin* 1993; **11**: 207–13.

3 Tsukada K, Tokunaga K, Iwama T, Mishima Y. The pH changes of pressure ulcers related to the healing process of wounds. *Wounds* 1992; **4**(1): 16–20.

4 Varghese MC, Balin AK, Carter M, Caldwell D. Local environment of chronic wounds under synthetic dressings. *Arch Dermatol* 1986; **122**: 52–7.

5 Leveen HH, Falk G, Borek B, *et al.* Chemical acidification of wounds: an adjuvant to healing and the unfavorable action of alkalinity and ammonia. *Ann Surg* 1973; **178**: 745–53.

6 Korting HC, Hubner K, Greiner K, *et al.* Differences in the skin surface pH and bacterial microflora due to the long term application of synthetic detergent preparations of pH 5.5 and pH 7.0. *Acta Derm Venereol* 1990; **70**: 429–57.

7 Sayegh N, Dawson J, Bloom N, Stahl W. Wound pH as a predictor of skin graft survival. *Curr Surg* 1988; **45**: 23–4.

8 Murahata RI, Toton-Quinn R, Finkey MB. Effect of pH on the production of irritation in a chamber irritation test. *J Am Acad Dermatol* 1988; **18**: 62–6.

Session 5:
CLINICAL EVIDENCE OF COST-EFFECTIVENESS

The role of cost-effectiveness analysis in woundcare

J POSNETT

YORK HEALTH ECONOMICS CONSORTIUM, UNIVERSITY OF YORK, UK

There will never be sufficient resources for the provision of health care, even health care of proven effectiveness, to all those who could benefit. In the face of such scarcity, it is inevitable that difficult choices have to be made. Cost-effectiveness analysis is a systematic means of comparing the relative costs and outcomes of available alternatives.

Evaluating cost-effectiveness

It is essential to consider both costs and patient outcomes when evaluating cost-effectiveness in woundcare. In a typical progression, a patient begins in an 'unhealed' state and may progress week by week into health states that are either better (typically 'healed') or worse (such as 'infected').

From the patient's perspective, the main goal of treatment is to maximize the number of weeks in the healed state. It follows that the main focus of patient outcomes is time to heal — the shorter the healing time, the more weeks in the healed state. Minimizing time to heal also helps reduce costs to the health care system. More significantly, it reduces the time a patient is exposed to the risk of progression into a more severe state, which can be both distressing and expensive. In some areas of woundcare (such as foot ulcers in diabetic patients) progression into more severe states can lead to hospitalization, amputation and even death.

If a new treatment alternative reduces time to heal at the same cost as the best existing practice, it is clearly more cost-effective. As the additional costs of the new treatment increase

EVIDENCE-BASED WOUNDCARE, EDITED BY A SUGGETT, G CHERRY, R MANI, W EAGLSTEIN, 1998.
INTERNATIONAL CONGRESS AND SYMPOSIUM SERIES NO 227 PUBLISHED BY THE ROYAL SOCIETY OF MEDICINE PRESS LIMITED

however, so its relative cost-effectiveness declines until a point is reached at which the additional costs involved in achieving better patient outcomes are judged to be too high. This does not imply that a more expensive treatment can never be cost-effective. Cost-effectiveness is not about saving money, it is about finding an appropriate balance between spending more and the value of improvements in outcome which result.

Some common themes

In undertaking or interpreting the results of a cost-effectiveness analysis in the woundcare field, there are a number of issues to consider. These include: time to heal, number of patients healed, rate of healing and rate of recurrence.

It is quite common for the results of a cost-effectiveness analysis to be expressed in terms of the average cost per healed wound (or per healed patient), but this can be misleading. Consider, for example, two treatments: both heal 75% of patients within 12 months and both have a zero rate of recurrence. If the number of patients healed is the outcome measure, both treatments are equivalent. If, however, the median time to heal is 10 weeks with treatment A and 25 weeks with treatment B, the results are deceptive. In most cases time to heal (or weeks in the healed state) is a more appropriate measure of outcome, and it is the incremental cost per additional healed week that is the relevant measure of cost-effectiveness.

Although time to heal is the primary focus of cost-effectiveness, information on the number of patients healed is also important in assessing the validity of a cost-effectiveness comparison. Consider, for example, a new treatment (treatment A) that reduces the mean time to heal from 12 weeks to five weeks. The average cost of treatment is £100 per week and the new treatment therefore saves £700 per patient (£100 × (12–5)). If the additional cost of the new treatment is £500 per patient, treatment A is clearly cost-effective compared with current practice. This claim is only valid, however, if 100% of patients are healed. Suppose both treatments heal 50% of patients after 12 weeks. The cost savings implicit in the new treatment are actually £350 per patient (£100 × 0.5(12–5)). Treatment A is then no longer unambiguously cost-effective.

Even if a clinical trial showed that 50% more patients were healed with treatment A than with current practice this is insufficient evidence on which to base an economic evaluation — more information on the time period of the trial is needed. Figure 1 shows typical healing curves for current practice, compared with a new treatment with a shorter median time to heal. Because the new treatment heals more quickly, the difference between the two treatments is maximized early in the period. A cost-effectiveness analysis which assumes that the difference in healing rates observed after, for example, 12 weeks is maintained to week 52, will considerably overestimate the potential benefits of the new treatment.

Finally, a superior treatment may generate more recurrent wounds in a given time period simply because it heals more quickly. Once a wound is healed it is at risk of recurrence and it is important to distinguish between the number of recurrences and the rate of recurrence. Reducing the rate of recurrence is important in terms of costs and patient outcomes — the number of recurrences is of little significance on its own.

Conclusions

Cost-effectiveness is always relative and invariably subjective. Whether the additional benefits of a new treatment are sufficient to offset the additional cost is typically a matter of judgement. The role of cost-effectiveness analysis is to ensure that, as far as possible, judgements are explicit and well-informed.

A review of cost-effectiveness in cavity wounds: clinical experiences in Japan using Allevyn Cavity wound dressing

N SHIOYA

WOUNDCARE HEALING CENTRE, KITASATO UNIVERSITY SCHOOL OF MEDICINE, TOKYO, JAPAN

A study was undertaken to evaluate the use of a hydrocellular foam dressing, Allevyn Cavity (Smith & Nephew) in cavity wounds. This presentation describes a secondary analysis of a subset of the original study data designed to evaluate the cost-effectiveness of Allevyn Cavity in relation to calcium alginate dressings.

Materials and methods

The study population comprised two groups of 36 patients from seven different hospitals with stage 3 or 4 pressure sores; all were treated with Allevyn Cavity dressings. This presentation will concentrate on the author's own study group, which consisted of 16 male and 20 female patients with a mean age of 68.6 years. Pressure sores were classed as stage 3 in 11 patients and stage 4 in 25 patients. All patients had underlying diseases including dementia (27.8%), other brain and nervous system disease (27.8%), Parkinson's disease (13.9%) and diabetes (11.1%). Wound sites included the sacrum (63.9%), the trochanter major (16.7%) and the heel (5.6%). Wound sizes were: mean length 6.6 cm (SD ± 3.4 cm), mean width 5.8 cm (SD ± 3.2 cm), and mean depth 1.4 cm (SD ± 1.0 cm).

EVIDENCE-BASED WOUNDCARE, EDITED BY A SUGGETT, G CHERRY, R MANI, W EAGLSTEIN, 1998.
INTERNATIONAL CONGRESS AND SYMPOSIUM SERIES NO 227 PUBLISHED BY THE ROYAL SOCIETY OF MEDICINE PRESS LIMITED

Most patients had been referred to the study group for plastic surgery, so the aim in most cases was to prepare the tissue for grafting. Consequently, time to spontaneous wound closure could not be used as an endpoint for cost-effectiveness evaluation. Frequency of dressing change was used instead. Efficacy was evaluated under two categories: effect on wound healing (A) and ease of use (B). These were subdivided into: effects on granulation, inflammation and pain (A) and ease of application and ease of removal (B). Subjective points ratings were awarded in each sub-category and pooled to give an overall score for each category. The average treatment period was 46.9 days (SD±19.3 days).

Results

Using the criteria described above, wound healing was rated as excellent in 25.9% of patients, effective in 25.9% and fair in 29.6%, with 81.5% of patients falling into one of these categories. The wound was unchanged in 1.1% and aggravated in 7.4%. The data were then broken down according to stage of pressure sore. In stage 3 patients (n=11), efficacy was rated as excellent in 27.3%, effective in 36.4%, fair in 0.0%, wound unchanged in 9.1% and wound aggravated in 27.3%. In stage 4 patients (n=25), the figures were 24.0%, 28.0%, 32.0%, 8.0% and 8.0%, respectively. Taking all patients together, ease of use was rated as very good in 16.7%, good in 44.4% and fair in 22.2%, with 83.3% of cases falling into one of these categories. Average frequency of dressing change was 3.1 days (SD±1.4 days).

Discussion

Measurement of cost-effectiveness is not a straightforward concept. In addition, the original study was primarily designed to evaluate efficacy. Therefore, to obtain an indication of relative cost-effectiveness, the results described above were compared with those from a study of calcium alginate dressings in 30 patients with stage 3 pressure sores[1]. Data from the two studies are compared in Tables 1 and 2.

Table 1 *Reduction in cavity depth for stage 3 pressure sores*

		Baseline	2 weeks	4 weeks	6 weeks
Alleyn Cavity wound dressing (n=22)	Average	12.2	10.0	7.7	6.9
	Improvement (%)	—	18.0	36.9	43.4
Calcium Alginate (n=30)	Average	9.9	7.9	7.4	5.3
	Improvement (%)	—	17.7	23.0	34.6

Table 2 *Frequency of dressing change in stage 3 pressure sores with Allevyn Cavity and calcium alginate dressing*

		Dressing change (times/case)	Frequency of dressing change (day)
Allevyn Cavity wound dressing (*n*=22)	Maximum	57	18
	Minimum	1	1
	Average	21.7	2.2
Calcium Alginate[1] (*n*=30)	Maximum	122	3.2
	Minimum	11	0.3
	Average	40.6	1.1

The average reduction in wound depth of stage 3 pressure sores treated with Allevyn Cavity after six weeks was 43.4%, compared with 34.6% for calcium alginate dressings. The average time between dressing changes for Allevyn Cavity was 2.2 days, compared with 1.1 days for the calcium alginate. These data suggest that Allevyn Cavity dressing is likely to be more cost-effective in pressure sore treatment than calcium alginate dressings.

Conclusion

The study found that Allevyn Cavity hydrocellular foam dressing is a useful addition to the products available for treating cavity wounds. Dressing change times can be extended through the use of this technology, and clinical acceptance in Japan is good.

Reference

1 Syotaro H, Nakanishi H, Kawabata N, *et al.* Clinical evaluation on SORBSAN (calcium alginate fiber dressing) for the treatment of skin ulcer. *JO Med Pharmaceutical Sci* 1994; **10**(2): 473–95.

A 100-patient cost-effectiveness trial of a hydrocellular and a hydrocolloid dressing

K HARDING

WOUND HEALING RESEARCH UNIT, UNIVERSITY OF WALES COLLEGE OF MEDICINE, CARDIFF, UK

A prospective, randomized, parallel group, 100-patient community-based clinical trial was undertaken to compare a hydrocellular dressing, Allevyn (Smith & Nephew) with an improved formulation hydrocolloid dressing. The primary objective was to define total dressing cost per patient over the eight-week treatment period, reflecting wound healing and dressing durability.

Methods and results

Many different wound types were recruited to the trial; 31% of all wounds were leg ulcers, 33% were pressure sores and 36% were classified as 'other wounds'. Every dressing change was assessed and all materials used were recorded, including retention dressings, saline solution and gloves. In order to accurately determine dressing durability, predetermined dressing change routines were eliminated and dressings changed only if there was leakage, imminent leakage or another clinical indication.

A total of 96 patients were evaluated for analysis under the following headings: durability, healing, cost-effectiveness, incidence of leakage, adverse incidents and patient comfort. After making efforts to maximize the length of wear of the dressing, durations (mean$\pm$SD) of 3.6$\pm$1.6 days and 4.1$\pm$1.6 days were noted for the Allevyn and hydrocolloid dressings respectively. This difference was not statistically significant. Table 1 describes the number of

EVIDENCE-BASED WOUNDCARE, EDITED BY A SUGGETT, G CHERRY, R MANI, W EAGLSTEIN, 1998.
INTERNATIONAL CONGRESS AND SYMPOSIUM SERIES NO 227 PUBLISHED BY THE ROYAL SOCIETY OF MEDICINE PRESS LIMITED

wounds in each wound category that were completely healed. Of the wounds treated, 46% of those treated with Allevyn and 33% of those treated with the hydrocolloid (p=0.045), were healed within the eight-week treatment period.

Cost data can be expressed in many ways: as cost per week, cost per patient and percentage of cost attributed to secondary dressing. Dividing the total cost of treatment for each product group by the number of patients completely healed gave a cost per healed patient of £130 for the Allevyn group and £179 for the hydrocolloid group. The major difference in cost per healed patient occurred in the pressure sore group; differences were less marked in the other two wound groups. To provide truly useful data, the cost of a treatment should be linked to its effectiveness. Nursing time was not considered as a cost, because of the difficulty of standardizing nursing practice in a community setting involving a large number of nurses.

The soiling of patient's clothes or bedclothes is an important issue in community care—elderly people living alone may have difficulty changing their sheets. The Allevyn group experienced a significantly lower incidence of leakage (p=0.037) and soiling (p=0.01). Seven patients (14%) in the hydrocolloid group were withdrawn due to adverse incidents which, in the opinion of the investigator, were due to the dressing. These incidents included maceration, pain and over-granulation. No adverse incidents were attributed to the use of Allevyn hydrocellular dressing.

Patients were asked to classify their dressings as either very comfortable, acceptable or uncomfortable. Although patient assessment of comfort is subjective, it is important. Comfort scores for Allevyn were significantly better than those for the hydrocolloid dressing (p=0.011).

Conclusion

The overriding concern in treating wound patients in the community is to achieve the best outcome for the patient. Cost-effectiveness is part of a complex equation that also considers

Table 1 *Number of wounds completely healed, following treatment with either Allevyn or a hydrocolloid dressing*

Leg ulcers	Allevyn	Hydrocolloid
Leg ulcers	2/16 (13%)	1/14 (7%)
Pressure sores	10/17 (59%)	4/15 (27%)
Other wounds	11/17 (65%)	10/17 (59%)
All patients	25/50 (46%)	15/46 (33%)

healing time and quality of life issues. Cost-effectiveness can be assessed in a variety of ways, but cost per healed patient is one valid measure. Nursing time is also a major component of treatment cost, and a dressing regimen that reduces the frequency of dressing changes, or allows patients or relatives to carry out the changes themselves, may be an important means of improving cost-effectiveness.

Cost-effective management of the diabetic foot

A FOSTER

KINGS COLLEGE HOSPITAL, DENMARK HILL, LONDON, UK

Diabetics make up approximately 2% of the general population but account for 50% of all leg amputations in the UK. Foot wounds are a major health problem for diabetic patients who have neuropathy, as they lose protective pain sensation and do not perceive trauma or infection to their feet. Neuroischaemic patients have both reduced pain sensation and a poor blood supply and cannot mount the inflammatory response needed to fight infection and to heal wounds. A small ischaemic foot ulcer that looks innocuous can rapidly extend and become gangrenous without effective care and this can lead to amputation, disability and death. Research shows that diabetic foot ulcers are very expensive to treat; it is very cost-effective if they are healed quickly and amputations prevented.

Wound management in the diabetic foot

The aims of management of the diabetic foot apply to the management of all wounds in all patients — to achieve rapid healing and prevent complications at minimum cost. Management should also be acceptable to the patient and disrupt normal life as little as possible.

Most multidisciplinary teams with a successful record in the management of diabetic feet agree that certain factors are essential if healing is to be achieved:

- neuropathic feet with plantar ulceration need pressure relief via special footwear and insoles
- critically ischaemic patients benefit from vascular intervention

EVIDENCE-BASED WOUNDCARE, EDITED BY A SUGGETT, G CHERRY, R MANI, W EAGLSTEIN, 1998.
INTERNATIONAL CONGRESS AND SYMPOSIUM SERIES NO 227 PUBLISHED BY THE ROYAL SOCIETY OF MEDICINE PRESS LIMITED

- all foot ulcers need regular debridement, cleaning, suitable dressing and infection control.

Prevention of ulceration is, in theory, achievable in most cases. Vulnerable patient groups need to be targeted for special help, and educational programmes are essential. Cost-effective management of foot wounds cannot be achieved without addressing these issues.

Ulcer care is expensive. Although the costs of individual dressings vary, a major part of the total cost is due to the salary of the staff who apply the dressing. Thus, in theory a dressing that does not need frequent changing is desirable. However in diabetic patients, in whom wounds need to be inspected for signs of deterioration, failure to change dressings regularly can be disastrous.

Within the NHS, health care trusts often pressurize health care professionals to cut costs — by reducing hospital visits, inpatient stays and the use of expensive antibiotics. This can often be achieved short term, but the long-term implications can include increased healing times and a rise in the number of amputations and deaths. An expensive episode of inpatient care may prove cost-effective, if it heals an ulcer which could have persisted for years and possibly resulted in a major amputation. The problem with considering short-term financial savings alone is that death can look alarmingly cost-effective.

Choosing a cost-effective dressing

A cost-effective dressing for the diabetic foot should be cheap, easy to apply, easily lifted for inspection and perform well within the shoe. There are many different dressings which, it is claimed, fulfil these criteria: two of these are Allevyn (Smith & Nephew) and Kaltostat (ConvaTec). The diabetic foot clinic at Kings College Hospital, London, carried out a randomized clinical trial to compare Allevyn with the alginate wound dressing, Kaltostat. These were considered in terms of ease of use — criteria of interest included speed of application, whether or not the dressing stayed in place in the shoe of an ambulant patient, ease of removal, absorbency, non-adherence, wound progress and patient comfort. Thirty patients were chosen and the randomization stratified according to ulcer type. The trial period was eight weeks or until the ulcer healed, whichever occurred first. Ulcers were assessed weekly but were redressed daily. Wound areas were traced at the start of the study and at weeks four and eight.

There was no significant difference in healing between the two products. Six patients improved in the Allevyn group and three in the Kaltostat group. Four patients had to be withdrawn from the Kaltostat group; in three cases, the dressing had plugged the wound preventing free drainage of exudate — one of these three patients developed severe cellulitis. No patients were withdrawn from the Allevyn group.

Conclusion

Allevyn was significantly easier to apply than Kaltostat and the time taken to apply it significantly shorter. Absorbency was better in the Allevyn than in the Kaltostat group. Lastly Allevyn was significantly easier to remove and less adherent to the wound. It is concluded that Allevyn is a cost-effective dressing for diabetic foot wounds.

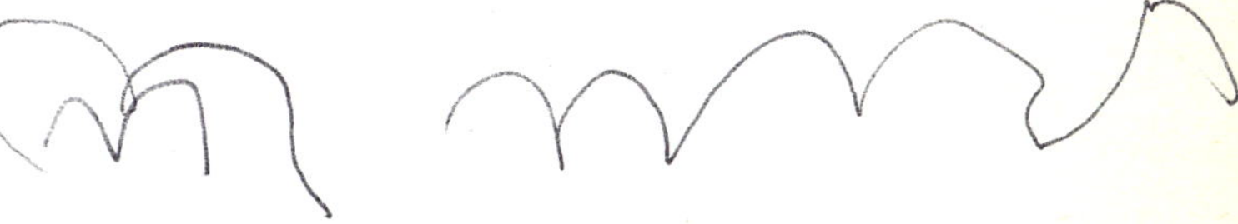

Session 6:
WOUNDCARE INTO THE MILLENNIUM

Evidence in wound management: what do we know and what do we think we know?

GW CHERRY

OXFORD WOUND HEALING INSTITUTE, DEPARTMENT OF DERMATOLOGY, CHURCHILL HOSPITAL, OXFORD, UK

Modern advances in biological research techniques at the molecular level have increased the gap between our understanding of the mechanism of wound healing and the clinical application of this knowledge[1,2].

A number of factors, in addition to the expansion of new knowledge, have contributed to this distance. The most important factor is probably that, in healthy individuals, tissue repair after acute injury is thought to occur at a maximal rate and is, in fact, not impaired unless adversely affected by localized or systemic conditions. In chronic wounds the underlying pathology contributing to impairment in healing must be identified and treated before the wound can begin to heal.

Woundcare can be traced back to early civilizations. In China, there is written history on wound management treatments dating back more than 1000 years. Some of the treatments described, such as animal fat-impregnated dressings, are still used in a modified form today—eg paraffin-embedded tulle grass. Many of the early treatments were based on the use of herbal remedies. The WHO estimates that 80% of the population still relies on plant-based medicines for their primary care[3] and there is a need for prospective, randomized controlled trials to assess whether or not these traditional wound healing therapies are effective (there are currently trials in progress in Vietnam).

There is considerable need for protocols for the care of different types of chronic wounds—such as leg ulcers, pressure sores and diabetic wounds. This need has been highlighted by the

EVIDENCE-BASED WOUNDCARE, EDITED BY A SUGGETT, G CHERRY, R MANI, W EAGLSTEIN, 1998.
INTERNATIONAL CONGRESS AND SYMPOSIUM SERIES NO 227 PUBLISHED BY THE ROYAL SOCIETY OF MEDICINE PRESS LIMITED

interest and support of the US FDA in setting up the Wound Healing Clinical Focus Group, with its mission to facilitate the development and assessment of products for wound healing. At a recent meeting held by this group, considerable discussion time was given to clinical-trial design issues for chronic cutaneous ulcers[(4)]. Other topics discussed were standard of care, discontinuation of study treatment due to adverse events, blinding, vehicle controls, wound assessment, endpoints and product sterility.

The National Pressure Ulcer Advisory Panel has also been instrumental in influencing policy in the management of pressure ulcers by basing its recommendations on supporting evidence[(5)]. This consists of:

- Positive results of two or more randomized controlled clinical trials on pressure ulcers in humans
- Positive results of two or more controlled clinical trials on pressure ulcers in humans or, where appropriate, positive results of two or more controlled trials in animals.

The newly formed European Pressure Ulcer Advisory Panel is following a similar evidence-based format in recommending different policy statements for the prevention and treatment of pressure ulcers.

Anecdotal comments on woundcare still carry considerable weight, meaning that the need for evidence-based research on standard treatments used in chronic wounds treatment, such as bandaging of venous ulcers, is even stronger[(6)]. There is also a need for the collation of such work, which is presently being performed by the Cochrane Wound Healing Group as well as various evidence-based medical journals[(7)].

Conclusion

The only way in which the gap between basic research and clinical application in wound healing can be narrowed is by increasing and promoting the use of evidence-based medicine.

References

1 Peacock EE Jr. Wound healing. In: Peters RM, Peacock EE Jr, Benfield JR, eds. *The scientific management of surgical patients.* Boston: Little Brown, 1983: 27–63.

2 Cherry GW, Hughes MA, Kingsnorth AN, Arnold FA. Wound healing. In: Morris PJ, Malt RA, eds. *The Oxford textbook of surgery.* Oxford: Oxford University Press, 1994: 3–23.

3 WHO Regional Office for the Western Pacific. *Research guidelines for evaluating the safety and efficacy of herbal medicines.* Manila: WHO, 1993.

4 FDA Dermatologic and Ophthalmic Drugs Advisory Committee Meeting 46, Wound Healing Discussion. Bethesda, Maryland, July 15 1997: 10–22.

5 Clinical practice guideline 15. *Treatment of pressure ulcers*. AHCPR publication 95–0652, 1994.

6 Cherry GW, Hofman D, Cameron J, Poore SM. Bandaging in the treatment of venous ulcers: a European view. *Ostomy/Wound Management* 1996; **42**(10A suppl): 13s–18s.

7 *Evidence-based medicine: linking research to practice* 1997; **2**(4): 97–128.

Wound management post-millennium

M STACEY

DEPARTMENT OF SURGERY, UNIVERSITY OF WESTERN AUSTRALIA, FREMANTLE HOSPITAL, AUSTRALIA

Many of the current aims and goals of research into wound healing will bear fruit some time after the beginning of the next millennium. These advances will aid progress towards the major goals of wound management, that is to achieve complete and more rapid healing of wounds and to maintain healing once it has occurred.

In broad terms, wounds will still be classified as acute and chronic and, within these major categories, will be separated into subgroups according to aetiology. It seems likely that the aims and goals for the care of different wound types will differ.

Acute wounds

The major acute wounds that present to clinicians are those caused by trauma and surgical intervention. Burns represent a specific subgroup of trauma.

Traumatic and surgical wounds

In wounds caused by either direct trauma or surgery, treatment will depend on the amount of tissue loss. The major focus of improved wound management will be to reduce the complications that occur in these wounds, which delay healing. The methods by which this can be achieved include greater adherence to the principles of wound hygiene and infection prevention, better postoperative or post-trauma pain control and better maintenance of tissue oxygenation. In addition to improving these principles of general management, there may be

EVIDENCE-BASED WOUNDCARE, EDITED BY A SUGGETT, G CHERRY, R MANI, W EAGLSTEIN, 1998.
INTERNATIONAL CONGRESS AND SYMPOSIUM SERIES NO 227 PUBLISHED BY THE ROYAL SOCIETY OF MEDICINE PRESS LIMITED

topical and/or systemic agents that can be added to wounds to enhance the speed and quality of healing. Such substances will be of great importance in tissues that currently heal very slowly — tendons, ligaments, bone and muscle for example — and may include tissue glues, chemoattractants for inflammatory cells, vasodilators, better analgesics and better antibacterial agents.

One further area in which simple major advances could be made — even today — is the widespread provision of moist wound healing products for minor injuries. In particular, minor household grazes, abrasions and cuts are currently treated with what could be regarded as archaic dressing methods and could be better treated with a wider availability of moist wound healing products. The onus is on the pharmaceutical companies to make these available and affordable to members of the community.

In major injuries resulting in significant tissue loss, the development of advanced tissue substitutes should revolutionize treatment. In particular, the use of epidermis, dermis, bone, cartilage, ligament and nerve replacements should become widespread and cost-effective. The development of non-immunogenic and disease-free human cell lines should enable such tissue substitutes to be available whenever required.

Burns

Major advances in burn management will also include the use of tissue substitutes, in particular dermal and epidermal substitutes, which would also be available on demand. These will almost certainly be used in combination with tissue glues and other factors that will enhance the growth of vessels into these substitutes. The net result will be that contractures should effectively be a thing of the past. Existing contractures could be simply treatable by excision and replacement with dermal and epidermal substitutes. For minor burns not requiring tissue replacement, the use of anti-scarring therapies will hopefully become widespread, and will almost certainly reduce the frequency and incidence of contractures.

Chronic wounds

The main chronic wounds seen in clinical practice are venous ulcers, diabetic foot ulcers and pressure ulcers. There are some similarities, but all have specific aetiological factors. The major focus in the future management of chronic wounds will be prevention. The mechanism for prevention will be different for each type of wound and incidence will, hopefully, be reduced. In addition, significant advances in the understanding of chronic wound healing should result in faster and more effective healing.

Venous ulcers

The major advances in reducing venous ulcer occurrence will be prevention of deep vein thrombosis as well as improved treatment of deep vein thrombosis, post-thrombotic damage and primary reflux of the deep veins. Identification of patients at risk will reduce the occurrence of deep vein thrombosis. This will include further identification of procoagulant states and more widespread use of prophylaxis in hospital patients and following injury. Improved methods of deep vein thrombosis prophylaxis and treatment will be developed. The methods for dissolving thrombi will be improved, to the point where deep vein thromboses can be completely dissolved, resulting in minimal or no damage to the valves within the deep veins. This will enable the vast majority of venous ulcers to be prevented.

In patients with venous ulcers who have either post-thrombotic damage from a previous deep vein thrombosis or primary venous incompetence, the management of the underlying problem should be greatly improved. With the advent of new bio-materials, synthetic vein segments could be developed, with an endothelial cell lining enabling good patency and function. These would be used to replace the major incompetent segments of the deep veins, therefore restoring competence to the calf muscle pump. In addition, treatment could be improved by better methods of compression that would actually assist the calf muscle pump and return its function to normal levels. In this way, the underlying problems that cause venous ulcers will be improved or corrected; this will result in a dramatic improvement in the ability of these wounds to heal.

Diabetic foot ulcers

The treatment of diabetes should hopefully be revolutionized with the advent of either better pancreatic or Islet of Langerhans transplants, or the induction of insulin secretion from other cells. Diabetes could become a disease that is either curable or that can be treated with minimal side-effects. The net effect of this will be the prevention of neuropathy, vascular disease, joint contractures, impaired vision and impaired immune response.

Diabetic foot ulcers would therefore be an uncommon clinical problem. For patients who presented with established diabetic foot ulcers, dynamic testing of pressure points should be greatly improved. The current methods that are employed to assess both the pressure points and methods of relieving pressure are primitive. With better pressure relief, prevention of calluses and subsequent ulceration would be greatly improved enabling better treatment for patients who did develop ulcers.

Pressure ulcers

The prevention of pressure ulcers should be improved by greater awareness of the problem, with better education of health professionals to identify patients at risk and more widespread use of better pressure-distributing mattresses and devices. Pressure ulcers would then be a rare problem in bedridden patients. In those patients whose ulcers are primarily due to disorders of, or damage to, peripheral nerves or the spinal cord, the neuropathy could be treatable by nerve transplants and nerve regeneration; this would probably be a more long-term aim than many of the other advances that have been described.

Chronic wounds options

For patients who develop chronic wounds the methods of treatment and evaluation will be greatly improved. The factors that are important in the healing process will be identified and there will be a better understanding of how these factors can be stimulated or inhibited within the wound, or added to the wound, in order to improve the healing process.

There will be two options for improving the healing of chronic wounds. One will be to radically debride chronic wounds and convert them to acute wounds and, with better management of the underlying problem, to speed up the healing process. The second option will be to treat the chronic wound itself with a variety of factors that will modulate the wound environment and return it to an active healing phase similar to an acute wound.

Healing state, modulation, evaluation and measurement

In addition to knowing more about the healing process and how to deal with the chronic wound, our knowledge on how to assess the wound should be greatly enhanced. It should be possible to assess the stage of healing of chronic wounds by assessments that may be performed directly on the wound, on wound fluid, on biopsies or on blood. From this information, we will be able to determine the likelihood of the wound to heal and, in addition, will be able to determine what is needed to achieve healing. This will enable specific treatments designed for the individual patient to be developed and prescribed.

The various methods of modulation of the healing process that may occur will include a number of possible levels of intervention. Deleterious agents that actually inhibit the healing process may themselves be blocked or inhibited by the addition of chemicals or biological substances. Factors that are known to actively stimulate the healing process may have their expression or activation up-regulated in the wound, either systemically or by topical applications. Refinements in the methods of topical application of active factors should ensure appropriate delivery for these to be effective in the wound.

There are a number of factors that impact on our evaluation of treatments that are used to heal wounds. The method of measuring healing may itself directly influence the results obtained in studies of clinical treatments. In the modern, cost-conscious health care environment it is extremely important to have an understanding of the cost-effectiveness of different treatments that are used to heal wounds. From the patient's perspective, the impact on quality of life of the wounds themselves, as well as the different treatments, is of major importance.

The methods used to evaluate healing will be better understood by those performing clinical trials in wound management. There will be a better understanding of the need to evaluate the clinical use of treatments to heal wounds in a different way than scientific studies that assess the influence that a specific agent has on the healing process. The major measure that will be used for clinical treatments will be complete healing of the wound using intention to treat analysis. Other measures such as size reduction during different time intervals will be used only to assess the effect of agents on the healing process, not their use in clinical practice.

In addition to measuring complete healing, it will also be important to measure recurrence of chronic wounds. This will also be part of the measurement process of any treatment method that is used in these patients.

Cost-effectiveness and quality of life

One of the major difficulties in assessing cost-effectiveness is the lack of an established method for determining it. Hopefully one method for different treatments, relating to both the individual and the health service, will be developed. This will be very important in determining the availability of new treatments.

It is likely that the impact on patients' quality of life will become a more prominent part of the evaluation of chronic wounds and chronic wound treatments. More focus should, in the future, be placed on understanding the importance of the consequences of having a chronic wound, such as strong and unpleasant odours, experiencing pain and having treatments that limit mobility, clothing, footwear and the ability to socialize. There will be many other wound-related factors that will be important in helping to improve patients' quality of life, some of which we will only appreciate as more quality of life studies are undertaken.

The factors that are identified will help in the development of different treatments that will, in part, be aimed at improving specific quality of life factors. This will then enable treatments to be individualized according to the factors that each patient identifies as important. The relationship between cost-effectiveness and quality of life will be further understood and a method of evaluating this and weighing up the different influences will be developed over a period of time.

Conclusion

As we proceed into the next millennium, the management of both acute and chronic wounds should be revolutionized. The advances will be different for the two types of wound. For acute wounds, a greater focus on the patient's systemic factors, modulation of potential complications in these wounds and application of active solutions to enhance normal healing will hopefully speed up the healing process. In addition, the use of tissue substitutes should revolutionize the management of both burns and other acute wounds where there is substantial tissue loss.

Chronic wounds should be less common because of the focus on prevention. For patients who do have established chronic wounds, evaluation should be able to assess the healing status of the wound, to assess the potential of the wound to heal and to identify the factors needed to improve healing. It would then be possible to better direct the specific treatment for that patient. The type of treatment should also incorporate factors that have been determined to provide the best quality of life for that individual patient and that are also most cost-effective.

Although some of these goals may seem idealistic, they are undoubtedly achievable. The outstanding question is how long into the next millennium it will take before most of these are achieved. It is also important to remember that many of these advanced treatments and developments will probably only affect the developed countries of the world; many of the treatments or dressings described are unlikely to be affordable in poorer countries and communities. It is therefore important that the broadening and improvement of training and education of health workers and patients — worldwide — must be reviewed as a priority as we proceed into the next millennium.

NOTES

NOTES